Ocean Innovation
Biomimetics Beneath the Waves

CRC Press Series in Biomimetics

Series Editor: Yoseph Bar-Cohen

Jet Propulsion Laboratory, California Institute of Technology

PUBLISHED TITLES:

Architecture Follows Nature—Biomimetic Principles for Innovative Design
Ilaria Mazzoleni

Biomimetics: Nature-Based Innovation
Yoseph Bar-Cohen

Ocean Innovation: Biomimetics Beneath the Waves
Iain A. Anderson, Julian F. V. Vincent, and John C. Montgomery

FORTHCOMING TITLES:

Natural Biophotonic Architectures: Complex Optical Effects and Bioimimetic Applications
Pramod Kumar and Kamal P. Singh

Mechanical Circulatory Support: Principles and Practice
Pramod Bonde

Ocean Innovation
Biomimetics Beneath the Waves

Iain A. Anderson
Auckland Bioengineering Institute, New Zealand

Julian F. V. Vincent
Institute of Marine Science and School of Biological Sciences,
New Zealand

John C. Montgomery
University of Bath, United Kingdom

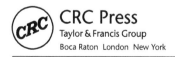

CRC Press
Taylor & Francis Group
Boca Raton London New York

CRC Press is an imprint of the
Taylor & Francis Group, an **informa** business

CRC Press
Taylor & Francis Group
6000 Broken Sound Parkway NW, Suite 300
Boca Raton, FL 33487-2742

First issued in paperback 2019

© 2016 by Taylor & Francis Group, LLC
CRC Press is an imprint of Taylor & Francis Group, an Informa business

No claim to original U.S. Government works

ISBN-13: 978-1-4398-3762-7 (hbk)
ISBN-13: 978-0-367-86526-9 (pbk)

Visit the Taylor & Francis Web site at
http://www.taylorandfrancis.com

and the CRC Press Web site at
http://www.crcpress.com

Sometimes we are lucky enough to know that our lives have been changed, to discard the old and embrace the new and run headlong down an immutable course...

It happened to me that summer's day when my eyes opened to the world beneath the surface of the sea.

Jacques Ives Cousteau [1]

Contents

Preface..ix

Authors..xiii

1 *Homo aquaticus* 1
   References   17

2 Swimming through syrup....................19
   References   36

3 The hydrostat 39
   References   54

4 Jet propulsion for soft bodies..................57
   Squid jet propulsion   57
   Jellyfish jet propulsion   62
   References   67

5 Buoyancy 69
   References   82

6 Drag...83
   Friction and form drag   83
   Wave drag   91
   References   95

7   Fins and brains **97**
    References   113

8   Listening to the silent world. **117**
    References   130

9   Underwater sensing for navigation and survival **133**
    Vision   133
    Scent   147
    Electrical and magnetic fields   149
    References   153

10   Stealth and show: A mind game. **157**
    References   175

Index **177**

Preface

There is something about the ocean that captures our imagination. What animals and plants live there? What do they look like? How do they breathe, move, see, and hear? How do they live and replicate? How do they survive being tossed around by the waves? How do they construct habitats to withstand the enormous forces of waves and currents? How do they know where they are and which way is up? We can certainly catch the creatures that live in the sea and examine them in the laboratory, but in many ways it is better to observe and study them in their natural surroundings. With recent advances in the technology of survival underwater we, as divers and researchers, can enter their world to learn how they have developed solutions to problems of existence that perhaps we can adopt for our own underwater exploration purposes. Given that life began in the ocean and that more than 80% of the Earth's surface is covered in water, it is ironic that we can dispatch probes to the edge of the solar system yet we have barely begun to explore deep ocean habitats and their spectacular diversity of life. Within the oceans, natural selection has been at work for millions of years. The great tree of life that Charles Darwin described "fills with its dead and broken branches the crust of the earth, and covers the surface with its ever branching and beautiful ramifications [2]."

This long sequence of experiments has produced both beautiful and bizarre examples of functional design, which have a real potential to inspire new technology. *Biomimetics* is the idea of creating new technology abstracted from what we find in nature. This book seeks that inspiration from the rich biodiversity of marine organisms.

Biomimetics from the ocean is not new: Alessandro Volta invented the electrochemical battery after working with electric rays (their biological name is *Torpedo*). In the final paragraph of his 1800 letter to the Royal Society titled: "On the Electricity excited by the mere Contact of conducting Substances of different Kinds" he refers to his battery as the *organelectrique artificial* [3]. Although he didn't use the word biomimetics he has been quoted as saying "nature has found the way to succeed with this in the electric organs of *Torpedo*" and that "we are not far from the possibility that our art could imitate them" [4]. Lord Cavendish, who gave his name to the Cavendish Laboratory in Cambridge, also drew inspiration from electric rays (Figures P.1 and P.2) [5]. If one marine organism, the *Torpedo* ray, could inspire the invention of the battery a little over 200 years ago, what other biomimetic inventions await discovery?

So, although the idea of biomimetics is not new, with the rapid progression in biological and engineering science, the potential for successful biomimetic technologies has never been greater. It is also true that as these disciplines have progressed, their practitioners have become increasingly specialized. Few of the biologists and engineers of today compare with the broadly curious natural scientists that Volta and Cavendish were in the eighteenth century. Recognizing this interdisciplinary need, the book brings both a biological and engineering perspective to the

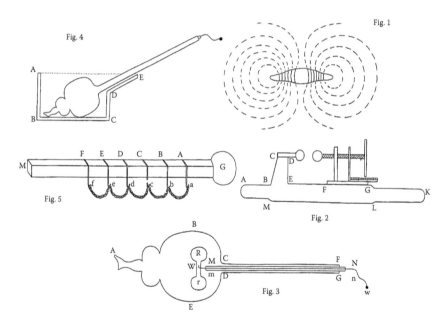

Figure P.1 Sketches by Lord Cavendish depicting his experimental equipment for exploring electric discharge from an artificial *Torpedo* ray [4]. In Fig. 1, he depicts a cross section of a ray body with dotted lines representing the "electric fluid." A device for measuring a spark discharge is depicted on the sketch labeled Fig. 2. His Fig. 3 sketch at the bottom, shows the artificial wooden *Torpedo* ray that was charged with electricity using capacitors (Leiden jars). In his paper, Lord Cavendish describes the electric shocks he received from the artificial *Torpedo* in air and fully immersed in a saltwater-filled trough (Fig. 4). A hand-held wooden electrode depicted in Fig. 5, which was touched to the *Torpedo*; electricity passed from the tin-filled head (G) through the brass chain to his thumb. (From Cavendish, H. *Philosophical Transactions of the Royal Society of London*, 1776. 66: 196–225 [4].)

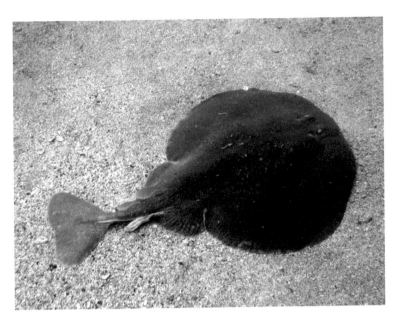

Figure P.2 Photograph of the blind electric ray (*Typhlonarke aysoni*). Electric rays use their electricity to stun their prey. They can also hold a significant charge. One of the authors (JCM) was fixing a specimen for histology that had been in formalin for about 20 minutes when he picked it up with forceps. The dead ray gave him a significant jolt—enough to drop the ray back into the fixative and throw the forceps across the room. (Photograph by Alison Perkins.)

biomimetic potential of ocean organisms. Each chapter explores an area where we as divers and technologists can benefit from understanding how ocean animals survive in the sea. Although our focus is on the potential use of biomimetics for ocean discovery, clearly, biomimetic technologies like batteries, possess utilities way beyond our ventures into the sea. We investigate questions that include What could we do usefully to make the aquatic world less alien to us? How can we effectively move about in a medium that is 1000 times denser than air? How can biomimetics be used to improve our diving and living?

While working on this book, our following expert colleagues have assisted us by voluntarily reviewing the chapters, and providing us with useful comments that have enabled us to improve the content and accuracy:

Promode Bandyopadhyay (Naval Undersea Warfare Center), Richard Bonser (Brunel University), John Cater (University of Auckland), Lily Chambers (University of Bristol), Richard Clarke (University of Auckland), Randall W. Davis (Texas A&M University), Lee Fuiman (University of Texas), Tony Hickey (School of Medical Sciences, University of Auckland), Ioannis A. Ieropoulos

(Bristol Robotics Laboratory), William M. Kier (University of North Carolina), Maarja Kruusmaa (Tallinn University of Technology), Akhlesh Lakhtakia (The Pennsylvania State University), David Moran (editor, *Dive New Zealand Magazine*), Raúl J. Martín Palma (Universidad Autónoma de Madrid), Julius J.B. Piercy (University of Essex), John Porrill (The University of Sheffield), Craig Radford (University of Auckland), Jonathan Rossiter (University of Bristol), Adam Summers (University of Washington), Laszlo Talas (University of Bristol), John J. Videler (University of Groningen), Steve Vogel (Duke University), and Shane Windsor (University of Bristol).

The authors gratefully thank them for their help! Through this book we share our own explorations of ocean innovation. We hope you enjoy it.

References

1. Madsen, A. *Cousteau—An Unauthorized Biography*. 1986, Trowbridge, Wiltshire: Redwood Burn Ltd.
2. Darwin, C. *Origin of Species and the Foundations of the Origin of Species*. 1859, St. Petersburg, Florida: Red and Black Publishers, ISBN 978-1-934941-45-4.
3. Volta, A. On the electricity excited by the mere contact of conducting substances of different kinds. In a Letter from Mr. Alexander Volta, F.R.S. Professor of Natural Philosophy in the University of Pavia, to the Rt. Hon. Sir Joseph Banks, Bart. K.B.P.R.S. *Philosophical Transactions of the Royal Society of London*, 1800. 90: 403–431.
4. Piccolino, M. The bicentennial of the voltaic battery (1800–2000): The artificial electric organ. *Trends in Neurosciences*, 2000. 23(4): 147–151.
5. Cavendish, H. An account of some attempts to imitate the effects of the *Torpedo* by electricity. By the Hon. Henry Cavendish, F.R.S. *Philosophical Transactions of the Royal Society of London*, 1776. 66: 196–225.

Authors

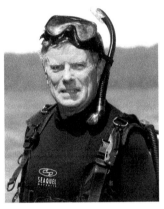

Iain A. Anderson is an associate professor with the Department of Engineering Science at the University of Auckland in New Zealand. He is also a cofounder of the Auckland Bioengineering Institute (ABI) where he is a principle investigator. He leads the ABI Biomimetics Laboratory which is exploring the use of dielectric elastomer electro-active polymers for stretchable electronics, wearable sensors, soft robots, and energy harvesters. Anderson is a keen advocate for fin propulsion. Together with his lab, he has developed and raced a fin-driven, human-propelled racing submarine. In 2012, with two of his former students he launched StretchSense Ltd. He is a director and chief scientist for this Biomimetics Lab spin-off company that produces soft and wearable sensors. As an avid underwater photographer, Anderson has written and illustrated a number of articles about life in the sea for magazines, including *Dive New Zealand Magazine* and *New Zealand Geographic*. He has also written and illustrated several books about sea life.

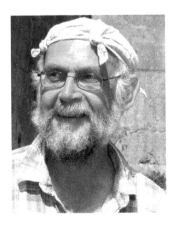

Julian F.V. Vincent is a zoologist. He earned his first degree at Cambridge University and second and third at Sheffield University. He started his career at the University of Reading as a zoologist and ended it at the University of Bath (both in the United Kingdom) as a professor of mechanical engineering. Vincent was part-time lecturer at the Royal College of Art & Design and Imperial College London until 2010. He has worked in many interdisciplinary contexts, such as mechanical engineering, materials science, architecture, design, creativity, biology, materials, food physics, and food texture. He is, and has been, a member of numerous scientific and advisory boards. He cofounded the Centres of Biomimetics in Reading and Bath and is president of the International Society for Bionic Engineering. Vincent is a Senior Research Associate in Zoology at Oxford University, Honorary Professor at the HochSchuele Rhein-Waal, and Adjunct Professor in Engineering and Materials at Clemson University.

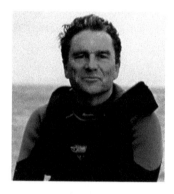

John C. Montgomery is a professor, and holds a personal chair in Biological Science at the University of Auckland. Until recently, he was the director of Auckland University's Leigh Marine Laboratory and its newly established Institute for Marine Science. His scientific work sits at the interface of marine science and neuroscience, and he has published extensively on sensory behavior and the physiology of fish, including hearing, hydrodynamic senses, and the quite extraordinary electrosensory system of sharks and rays. The neuroscience context of his work includes the consideration of central mechanisms to distinguish signals and noise in sensory input and the evolution of the cerebellum. Montgomery's work has been recognized by his election to the Royal Society of New Zealand, an International Brain Research Organization Fellowship, a Fulbright Scholarship, and most recently a James Cook Fellowship from the Royal Society of New Zealand. He also plays an active role in promoting marine science and communicating science to the public.

Chapter 1 *Homo aquaticus*

Will we ever be able to live and move about effortlessly beneath the surface of the sea without the need for cumbersome SCUBA (Self-Contained Underwater Breathing Apparatus)? Jacques Cousteau (1910–1997), the underwater explorer and cinematographer, and coinventor of the underwater demand regulator, predicted the emergence of a new class of a technologically augmented human. *Homo aquaticus* would be able to swim to depths of a mile and be capable of inhaling water, just as a fish does, with mechanical assistance to extract oxygen from the water [1]. Cousteau predicted that this would be a reality within 50 years. Fifty years have passed and his prediction has not come true. Some progress has been made and while we are closer to realizing this goal much work remains. Ideas are required and for these we look to the ocean's inhabitants for inspiration.

One can get a momentary and brief appreciation of what it would be like to realize Cousteau's vision while free diving on a single breath of air; but unfortunately the time below is short. In 2012, the New Zealand free diver William Trubridge descended to 125 m in the Bahamas without fins or other mechanical assistance, a World Record attempt that was disallowed because he failed the surface protocol—to remove his goggles and signal that he was OK. This judgment lapse was perhaps either due to the reduction in oxygen or to the buildup of carbon dioxide in his tissues and blood. Breath-holding abilities as those seen in athletes such as Trubridge can be learned and improved through training and exercise [2] but for most of us, depth and time are limited to a dozen meters or less and for durations of less than a minute.

Using ballast to get the diver down and an inflated suit for ascent enables a competing free diver to reach greater depths than Trubridge: about 3.5 minutes for a round trip [2]. But when physical exertion is required and the diving is repetitive our breath-holding capabilities are severely curtailed. For the Ama pearl divers of Japan and South Korea, who dive in much shallower water, the duration for repetitive free diving is typically 30 seconds with half of this on the bottom, after which the Ama diver rests on her float for about 30 seconds while she takes some deep breaths [2]. This is much less than some aquatic mammals that are of similar size or bigger than us. Among the most extreme pinniped divers (e.g., seals, sea lions, and walruses) are the elephant seals that can remain at sea for months foraging and migrating. It is while at sea that they display extreme diving capabilities. Northern elephant bull seals (*Mirounga angustirostris*) from San Miguel Island in California have been observed diving continuously at sea, submerged for 86% of the time at depths averaging about 388 m with the deepest dives between 1 km and over 1.5 km [3]. Sperm whales (*Physeter macrocephalus*) have been observed

1

to dive for 40–50 minutes and visit depths of 400–1200 m [4]. Not only do these remarkable animals withstand a lack of oxygen and high levels of carbon dioxide but also survive immense pressures. It is clear that we are not born with the same capabilities and in order to realize Cousteau's prediction any time soon, we must seek ways to augment our abilities through technology.

For actively swimming humans to endure being submerged more than a minute requires a SCUBA device. This usually consists of a demand regulator coupled to a cylinder of compressed air or mixed gases, if submerged at great depths or for extended periods (Figure 1.1). A scuba diver who has been breathing air at depth requires the air to be delivered at a pressure equal to the surrounding water, and as this pressure increases, the partial pressure of oxygen also rises. As the oxygen partial pressure approaches 2 atmospheres (about 1/5 of the air we breathe is oxygen so that at 10 atmospheres pressure, approximately 100 m depth, the oxygen partial pressure will be 2 atmospheres), the oxygen itself becomes toxic, so for very deep diving the proportion of oxygen must be closely controlled. This is a problem for "technical" or commercial diving, as sports divers rarely if ever go to such depths.

At all depths, nitrogen dissolves into our tissues (especially in fat) and the nitrogen concentration increases with both depth and time. When the diver returns to the surface of the sea the nitrogen has to escape, but this takes time. Without

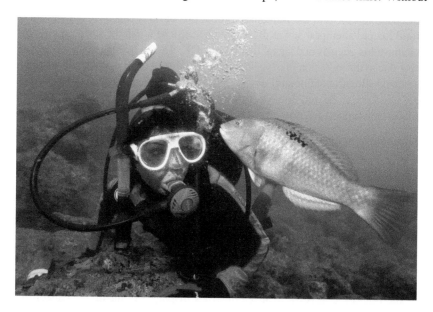

Figure 1.1 A diver breathing through a demand regulator mouthpiece attached to a compressed air cylinder encounters a small spotted "Spotty" wrasse (*Notolabrus celidotus*) in Matheson's Bay, New Zealand. Surprisingly, it is not frightened by the bubbles and noise from the diver's regulator. (Photo by Iain A. Anderson.)

staged "decompression" stops, the nitrogen might come out of solution forming small bubbles within the body. These often painfully lodge within the joints in a sometimes fatal condition called the *bends*. The bubbles can also form within the brain and spinal cord resulting in neurological damage.

The bends can be avoided by a slow and staged return to the surface and the use of gas mixtures that substitute nitrogen with smaller molecule inert gases such as helium that are rapidly cleared from tissues. Bubble-free rebreather technologies are also available. Rebreathers still require mixed gases at depth, and also recirculate the exhalant gas through a scrubber to remove CO_2 and inject oxygen into the mix to replace that taken up in the lung. Whales and seals avoid the nitrogen problem mainly because the alveoli in their lungs can collapse at a relatively shallow depth, typically in the first 50–100 m for most marine mammals [5], and therefore the concentration of nitrogen in their tissue cannot become saturated.

It follows that with repeated shallow diving it is possible that marine mammals can get the bends. For instance, extreme divers like the beaked whales might alter their behavior if a predator like the orca is around, from deep to repetitive shallow diving. If alveoli are not collapsed at shallow depths then nitrogen will continue to dissolve in their tissue at a relatively high rate. It has been suggested that human sonar, mistaken for the sounds of the orca, might encourage this shallow diving behavior thus leading to nitrogen saturation in the tissue and the bends, and that this might explain some whale beachings [6].

It is obviously the gas that we bring with us when SCUBA diving which is the cause of the problems, but we must breathe air that is 20% oxygen. Since the oceans are full of oxygen, why not breathe the oxygen dissolved in seawater? Why can't we at least partially realize the dream of Cousteau? Attempts during the past 60 years to make an underwater breathing chamber, or artificial gill have met with mixed success. The fundamental challenge is that although oxygen is abundant in seawater, the density of dissolved free oxygen is low: its mass in surface water (7.4 g/m^3) is only about 3% of the oxygen within an equal volume of the air above the sea (250 g/m^3).

Until recently, the only way to extract oxygen was by diffusion, a slow process governed by concentration differences. At our basal metabolic rate we consume oxygen at about 0.24 liters/min [7], to maintain tissue function throughout the body. Therefore, if we were to consume all the free oxygen in filtered water we would need about 8 liters/min of water*; quite feasible. Respiration in air is governed more by removal of carbon dioxide rather than the oxygen supply, but in terms of aquatic respiration, it is harder to obtain oxygen than to remove carbon dioxide; accordingly, oxygen supply forms the focus for our discussion.

---

* The density of air is 1.225 g/liter so oxygen density is 0.2 times this or 0.245 g/liter. So, we require 0.24 liter/min × 0.245 g/liter = 0.06 g/min. With 0.0074 g/liter of oxygen in water, we have 0.06 g/min/0.0074 g/liter = 8.1 liters/min.

The real challenge is extracting oxygen from the water using diffusion alone. Some pioneers have produced an artificial gill to accomplish this. One of the first documented artificial gill devices was demonstrated during the early 1960s by W.L. Robb, an engineer with General Electric, who was investigating the properties and uses of silicone membranes. In one of his experiments, he placed a 30 g hamster underwater in a cubic chamber 1 ft (0.3 m) across lined with a silicone membrane of a total area of 3 square feet (0.28 m²) and circulated freshwater past the membrane walls fast enough (about 38 liters/min) for adequate gas exchange [8]. The idea was simple: as oxygen (O_2) was consumed by the hamster, the partial pressure of this gas would go down within the chamber. The concentration gradient across the silicone membrane, in accordance with Fick's First Law (Figure 1.2), resulted in the diffusion of oxygen across the membrane into the chamber. Similarly, respiratory carbon dioxide (CO_2) produced by the hamster diffused through the membrane into the water. Robb estimated that his gill could remove about 5% of dissolved oxygen from water.

A square box is not an ideal geometry for oxygen extraction. If we could surround the same volume of gas with a long and narrow tube we would get a much greater

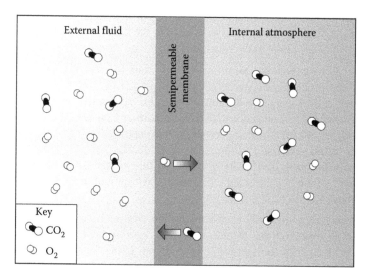

Figure 1.2 Section of a semipermeable wall. Oxygen (O_2) depletion within results in an oxygen flux from the external fluid to the internal atmosphere of the box. Carbon dioxide (CO_2) diffuses the other way. It is governed by Fick's First Law that describes the movement of a solute such as a dissolved gas from a region of high concentration to one of low concentration: $J = -DA(dC/dx)$ where J is the diffusion flux (amount of material per unit area in a given time), D is a constant, A is the cross-sectional area, C is the concentration of a substance (e.g., O_2 or CO_2 in this case), and x is the position. (Drawing by Vivian L. Ward.)

surface-to-volume ratio. This was the basis for the artificial gill developed by Waldemar Ayres (described in *Popular Mechanics* [9]). On August 6, 1962, Ayres tested the concept at Jones Beach, New York, using a hose made of multiple 25 m long floating tubes connected together and to a mouthpiece in a closed circuit. A nonreturn valve ensured that exhaled air passed along the full length of tubing before returning to the mouthpiece. Gas was exchanged with the water across a membrane on the submerged side of each tube. A picture from the *Popular Mechanics* article depicts Ayres sitting in the shallows with his upper body out of the water while breathing through the apparatus. Ayres maintained respiration for an hour and a half, until the tube flooded; this was perhaps the first demonstration of a human gill-like gas exchange device. His patent [10] drawing depicts a wearable underwater gill that is substantially more compact than the working prototype he tested in the shallows. While Ayres demonstrated what was possible, he also highlighted the substantial further development required to make an artificial gill a practical and wearable device.

In the 1980s, E.L. Cussler and his colleagues at the University of Minnesota boosted the cross-sectional area for gas diffusion in a tube gill by using gas exchange modules composed of thousands of 22 cm long, 200 μm wide (internally), 25 μm thick microporous polypropylene fibers held tightly together into a small volume that was flushed with fresh water [11]. When oxygenated water was forced over the tubes, oxygen exchanged into the tubes and carbon dioxide was removed. A gill that could support a hamster was demonstrated. Forty of the hamster-sized modules used together were able to provide adequate gas exchange for a small dog, although the dog-sized lung was too small for a human.

These proof-of-concept studies demonstrate that an artificial gill can provide metabolic gas exchange with water at life-sustaining levels by making contact with as much water as possible through a large surface area of semipermeable material (e.g., a large enclosure or numerous small tubes). The challenge is to extract oxygen from the water, at a rate that can sustain human life.

One could imagine using many more gill tubes with smaller diameters and thinner walls and packing more of them together. Air, like water, is viscous and for narrower tubes frictional effects increase. If we reduce the radius of each tube by half each would only carry 1/16 the flow for the same pressure difference.* While this would increase the surface area for diffusion, as tubes become narrower and

---

* This phenomenon is described using Poiseuille's equation, which relates the flow rate Q to the pressure difference ΔP along a tube of radius R and length L for an incompressible fluid of viscosity μ with a volumetric flow rate of Q:

$$\Delta P = Q\frac{8\mu L}{\pi R^4}$$

It is assumed that the fluid is incompressible, the flow is laminar, and it is traveling through a pipe of constant circular cross section.

more numerous, it would become increasingly difficult to inhale and exhale, and therefore drive air through the system. It would also become increasingly difficult to pass water around the narrow tubes.

Living sponges have a design solution to this problem. Water that carries plank-tonic food to the sponge enters a sponge's external openings and travels along fine internal passages (ostia) to chambers lined with choanocytes, cells that beat the water with flagella and drive the flow (Figure 1.3). There is a huge growth in cross-sectional area between ostia and choanocyte chambers so that the water flow slows down substantially and food is trapped and ingested by choanocytes. The exhaust water then passes through larger exhalant passages into a central cavity and then departs the sponge through the osculum. Henry M. Reiswig at McGill University [12] calculated the relative speed of water flow at different points in the system by determining the total cross-sectional area that the water must flow through at different levels. For one species of the "amorphous" Western Atlantic sponge (*Haliclona permollis*), water enters the ostia at 0.57 mm/s, but once inside the choanocyte chamber the velocity slows 100-fold! However, the exhaust water then accelerates and exits the osculum at 10 times the speed at the start, perhaps helping to flush it away.

We can apply this example to the design of an artificial gill. As water is incom-pressible, we could deliver water through a large pipe (fast flow) that is connected to a manifold opening into numerous small pipes with a greatly increased total tube cross-sectional area. Here, the flow velocity will reduce, increasing the time for gas exchange to occur, and the water will come into contact with an increased surface area for diffusion. The tubes, that can be made shorter, then drain into larger pipes with significantly less resistance to flow. A concise way of describing this design principle is to have numerous "small pipes at exchange sites and large pipes for moving fluid from one exchange site to the other" [14, p. 57].

We could consider a vast array of small gas transfer pipes all packed together and facing a tidal current. Although impractical for the diver, this could function as a gas transfer station for an underwater habitat. Perhaps we could fabricate this as a giant porous underwater sock—reminiscent of a wind sock. It might resemble the sock-like salp (Figure 1.4), whose skin contains hundreds of water-filtering zooids that collectively present a huge surface area to the water.

Using skin for gas exchange is universal in the animal world: all animals exchange gas through their skin to a greater or lesser extent—including humans. While most tissues rely totally on the arterial blood oxygen supply, living cells within our skin can directly exchange gases with the air: approximately 1% of our oxygen supply comes through the skin, and the cells in the outer 0.25–0.4 mm of skin are supplied directly from air [15]. For smaller animals, including many amphibians such as frogs and lizards, a large fraction of oxygen and carbon dioxide diffuses through their skin [16], and reptile scales are not an impediment to gas exchange.

(a)

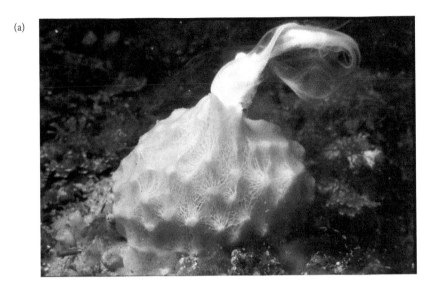

(b)

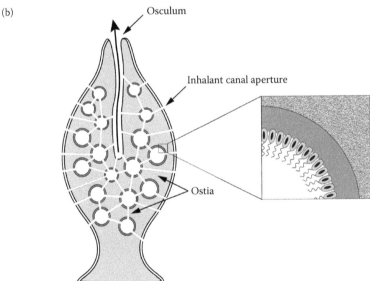

Figure 1.3 (a) A golf ball sponge (*Tethya fastigiata*) at the Poor Knights Islands (New Zealand). One of the authors (IAA) squirted a milk solution into the sponge's exhaust aperture (osculum). The pumping action of the many choanocytes is evident with the backflow of the milk that is visible. (Photo by Iain A. Anderson.) (b) Sponge schematic depicting the passages (ostia) between the choanocyte-lined chambers and a close-up of one of the chambers. (After Hentschel, U. et al. *Nature Reviews Microbiology*, 10(9), 641–654, 2012 [13].) (Redrawn by Vivian L. Ward.)

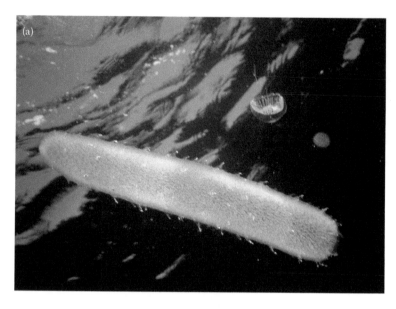

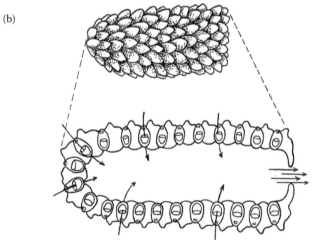

Figure 1.4 (a) A salp colony (possibly *Pyrosoma atlanticum*) drifting past the Poor Knights Islands (New Zealand), approximately 200 mm long is lit up by the photographer's flash. (Photo by Iain A. Anderson.) (b) The skin of this colony is home for many hundreds of zooids actively pumping water while filtering planktonic food and exchanging metabolic gases. (Drawing by Annelise Wiebkin.)

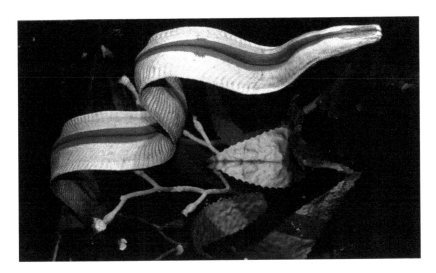

Figure 1.5 Yellow-bellied sea snake (*Pelamis platura*). While submerged, over 20% of its oxygen demand can be met by gas exchange through the skin. The yellow-bellied sea snake inhabits tropical waters from the east coast of Africa to the west coast of the Americas. This captive specimen that strayed into much cooler New Zealand waters was being nursed back to health in an aquarium. (Photo by Iain A. Anderson.)

The yellow-bellied sea snake (*Pelamis platura*) (Figure 1.5) gets up to 22% of its oxygen through the skin, which significantly extends its breath-holding time [17]. Imagine a "gill suit" that supplements our underwater air supply. Developments in the fabrication of structured or meta-materials might turn this into a reality: replacing the open cell foam of neoprene (a common material used in the manufacture of diver's wetsuits and drysuits) with an open porous gas exchange foam material that supplements the air supply. Of course, if gas can be exchanged with water then heat can also be lost; another design challenge!

Returning to the tube-gill system: water that is adjacent to the tube-gill membrane's surfaces will contain less oxygen, due to retention of a boundary layer. Unless stirred, gas diffusion will be impaired (Figure 1.6). The choanocytes within a sponge avoid this issue as they drive the flow using their flagella, which stirs the water in the choanocyte chamber. Water mixing improves the likelihood of trapping food, and decreases the diffusion distance by bringing fresh oxygen-rich water up against the diffusion surface. This idea has applications directly to microfluidics. Microarrays of artificial cilia have been proposed as a means for fluid transport, but they can also mix a fluid at the microscale and this can enhance diffusion. These can operate on electrostatic principles [18,19]. Artificial cilia could also be used for micromixing as an aid to improved diffusion. Issues associated with pushing fluids at low speeds and over such short distances are discussed further in Chapter 2.

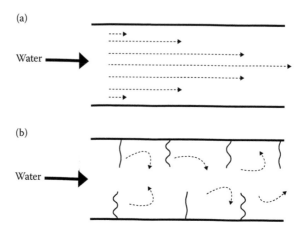

(a)

Water

(b)

Water

Figure 1.6 We depict (a) water flowing between plates or in a tube. If the flow is laminar there will be little mixing within the fluid cross section. This results in an oxygen-depleted zone near the walls that effectively increases the diffusion distance there so that the net flux of gas will be reduced. If cilia-like mechanisms could be placed along the walls (b) they could be used not only to drive the flow but also to stir it so as to encourage mixing across the fluid cross section, thus effectively reducing the diffusion distance, and enhancing gas diffusion. (Drawing by Iain A. Anderson.)

No matter how well we mix water above the membrane, we still cannot reduce the diffusion distance to less than the thickness of the membrane, unless we get rid of the membrane altogether. This is what many freshwater insects do. The saucer bug (*Aphelocheirus*) has developed a different way of keeping the water at a distance without a membrane. Tiny bristles that are spaced close enough over the insect's body provide support for the air–water interface. This immediately solves the problem with the efficiency of diffusion: it is now as effective as it can be because there is no longer a membrane in the way. Another way to promote gas exchange directly with air and with no membrane in this way is by bubbling the air up through the fluid (Figure 1.7).

Perhaps we will never be able to extract all the gas we need to sustain human metabolism underwater. But there might be an opportunity to at least supplement the gas supply we carry with us. Imagine a modified rebreather that obtains some of its oxygen from the surrounding water using a gill-like mechanism for direct gas exchange with water. What other design features can we bring to this challenge?

For clues we can focus on how a fish's gill works (Figure 1.8). Oxygen moves from the water into the gill by simple diffusion. Once there, it is carried away by the blood stream, attached to the hemoglobin in the red blood corpuscles. The rate of diffusion will be related to the difference in concentration of oxygen

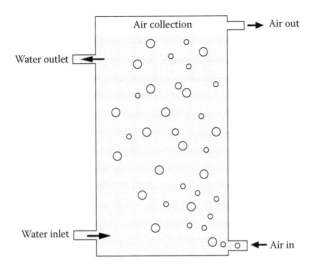

Figure 1.7 No membrane is needed if we simply bubble exhaust air through water. The diffusion area is effectively the combined surface area of all bubbles and we have discarded the restriction of the membrane. And if the bubbles are really small and there are many of them then the surface for gas diffusion will be huge. (Drawing by Vivian L. Ward.)

in the water and in the blood, and the distance along which it has to diffuse. Therefore, the membrane (epithelium) between the blood and the seawater should be as thin as possible, and the oxygenated blood should be removed from the gill as quickly as possible allowing oxygen-poor (deoxygenated) blood to take its place. The deoxygenated hemoglobin that is carried in the red cells has a high affinity for oxygen. In addition, oxygen binding to hemoglobin is "cooperative" in that as the first of four oxygen molecules bind to hemoglobin each additional molecule becomes easier to bind. This is further facilitated by changes in pH, as hemoglobin generally has a much greater affinity for oxygen at an alkaline pH. At the gills, carbon dioxide is also released by hemoglobin and the blood, and this diffuses into the water. As carbon dioxide leaves the blood through the gills, the pH in the blood rises and this improves the affinity of hemoglobin for oxygen. Overall, the efficient mopping up of oxygen by hemoglobin acts as an oxygen sink on the blood side of the membrane and this helps to drive diffusion. In tissues, oxygen concentrations are very low and carbon dioxide produced through respiration drives down pH. Hemoglobin then switches from a sink to an oxygen source in oxygen-poor, more acidic tissues. This greatly enhances diffusion gradients, and is a system that is clearly worth mimicking.

Of course, a fish gill transfers oxygen from liquid to liquid; water to blood. For our lungs, a two-module system would be required: one for taking up the oxygen from water and another for releasing the oxygen into inspired air. Such a system

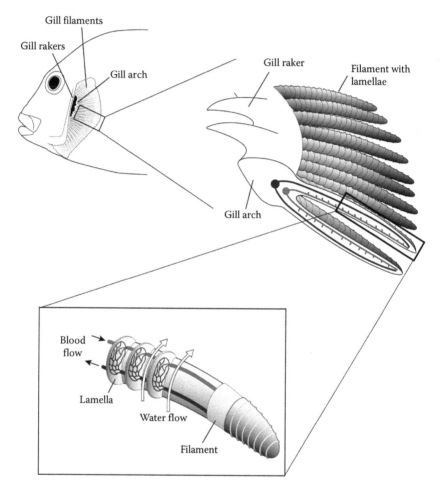

Figure 1.8 Schematic of a fish gill. Blood entering the gill (afferent blood vessel) is low in O_2. The blood passes through the capillary network to another vessel that leaves the gill (efferent blood vessel). The water travels along the outside of the gill in the opposite direction to the capillary blood, an example of countercurrent flow. (Drawing by Vivian L. Ward.)

has been trialed by researchers in Japan with an oxygen carrier solution being pumped from one interface to the other (Figure 1.9). The membrane modules contained numerous polypropylene or polyolefin hollow fibers that were typically 330 μm in diameter with 30 μm thick walls. Several oxygen carriers have been tried using this setup and these include bovine hemoglobin [20]. The researchers also harnessed a well-known temperature effect common to most mammalian hemoglobins. Hemoglobin oxygen affinity generally increases in cold and

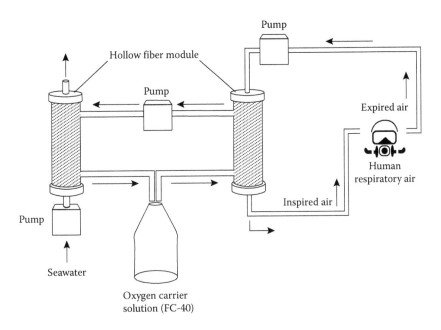

Figure 1.9 This schematic shows how an oxygen carrier solution can be used within an artificial gill. Seawater is pumped through the hollow fiber module on the left, and gas exchange takes place between the pumped seawater and an oxygen carrier solution. The pumped carrier solution passes through another hollow fiber module on the right where oxygen is released into air that is inspired by the diver. (After Nagase, K.-I., Kohori, F., and Sakai, K. *Journal of Membrane Science*, 215(1–2), 281–292, 2003 [20].) (Drawing by Vivian L. Ward.)

decreases in warm blood.* By using the temperature sensitivity of hemoglobin at 20°C oxygen is easily bound, and then released at 37°C. Mimicking hemoglobin's oxygen uptake and release capacity could make a human-sized gill feasible [20]. Other oxygen carriers could be used for this, such as perfluorocarbons [21]. Perfluorocarbons are organic molecules in which the hydrogens have been replaced with halogens, usually fluoride, which have been used successfully, in the clinical environment, for liquid ventilation of patients with lung ailments [22]. They have some interesting properties in this regard including high solubility of oxygen and carbon dioxide, and low surface tension. One of the obvious drawbacks of this scheme compared to Ayre's simple breathing driven diffusion tube lung is the requirement for fluid pumping of the oxygen carrier, pumping of the

---

* Note that this property is a major issue in most mammals when they become hypothermic as hemoglobin will less easily release oxygen to tissues. Although cold tissues require less oxygen due to depressed metabolic rates, numerous mammals (e.g., reindeer and cetaceans) appear to have evolved hemoglobins that are less affected by temperature in order to supply oxygen to peripheral tissues.

seawater, and of the air. Mechanical assistance to overcome the inertia of moving such a dense liquid into and out of our lungs would also be required. There is clearly no obvious way to use perfluorocarbons in a passive system that is driven by the diver's own chest muscles.

Returning to the fish gill: as water flows over, from front to back, one might expect that the deoxygenated blood should flow in the same direction, so that when blood and water meet, on opposite sides of the gill epithelium, there is a maximal difference in oxygen content. But this difference would soon tail off across the gill lamella, such that oxygen would not diffuse into the blood toward the back of the lamella because the concentration gradient would have disappeared.

This is not what happens. Instead, the gill works as a countercurrent exchange mechanism (Figure 1.8), in which the liquids (arterial blood and water) run in opposite directions. Countercurrent systems are found throughout biology and technology (e.g., fish gills, refrigeration, air conditioning, chemical plants, etc.), where a solute or heat is being transferred from one fluid (liquid or gas) to another.

In countercurrent exchange, the maximum gradient is smaller but is more constant, so that the seawater leaves the gill with more of the oxygen removed from it. Fish gill arches also have rakers, bony protrusions that protect the fragile gills from particles that can cause mechanical damage, and control the direction of water flow across the lamellae, ensuring that there is maximal exposure of water to the exchange surfaces.

Hence, the gill chamber has a number of functions, not just protecting the gills (which are very fragile) from dirt (which can sit in the gaps between the gill lamellae) or mechanical damage, but controlling the direction of flow across the lamellae, and ensuring that as much water as possible is directed across them.

There is, however, at least one further trick from fish that may be of use to us. This is the countercurrent exchange multiplier, based on the principal of countercurrent exchange but used for concentrating a substance instead of just transferring it (Figure 1.10). Bony fishes can harness specialized hemoglobins that are highly pH sensitive. These are used to secrete oxygen from the blood stream into the swim bladder (the swim bladder is the fish's equivalent of the buoyancy compensator used by divers). Oxygen-rich arterial blood enters a special network of blood vessel loops (rete mirable). Oxygen unloads from the hemoglobin as it passes through the gas gland due to the secretion of lactic acid. This is known as the Root effect (named after its discoverer R.W. Root) where acid pH not only reduces the affinity for hemoglobin to carry oxygen but also reduces its oxygen-carrying capacity. The Root effect hemoglobin may also have evolved to increase oxygen supply to other tissues [22], but within the countercurrent exchanger their role is to increase the concentration of oxygen in the blood leaving the gas gland. As the "venous" blood then passes back through the exchanger it has a higher oxygen concentration than the incoming arterial blood. Therefore, more oxygen diffuses

(a)

Swim bladder

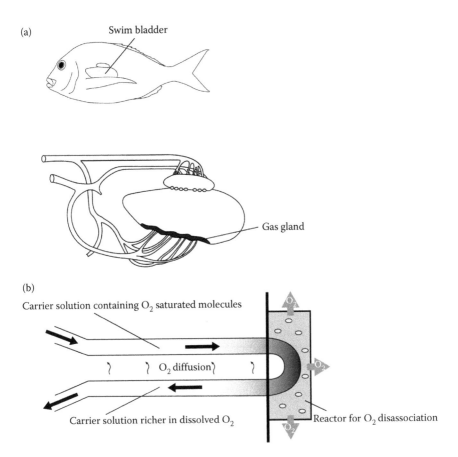

Gas gland

(b)

Carrier solution containing O_2 saturated molecules

O_2 diffusion

Carrier solution richer in dissolved O_2

Reactor for O_2 disassociation

Figure 1.10 (a) Schematics of the fish swim bladder that lies in the gut cavity just below the vertebral column. The gas gland is often visible as a red patch on the surface of the swim bladder. It provides for the secretion of gases from the blood to the swim bladder. There is usually a separate section of the swim bladder that can be opened or closed to the main bladder. This section provides for gas reabsorption if the swim bladder is overinflated. (Drawing by Vivian L. Ward.) (b) Countercurrent multiplier mechanism: Acid secretion from the gas gland causes oxygen to be released from the hemoglobin. So the blood returning through the venous capillary now has a very high concentration of oxygen that diffuses across to the incoming pathway. Thus, the oxygen concentration within the gas gland grows, culminating in the release of gas from the circuit to the bladder. (Drawing by Iain A. Anderson.)

across into the arterial blood, which then passes into the gas gland, releasing more oxygen into solution. In this way, the countercurrent exchange multiplier steadily builds up the acidity and oxygen concentration until oxygen bubbles off into the swim bladder. A synthetic countercurrent exchange multiplier such as this could potentially provide a low-pressure mechanism for collecting gas underwater, perhaps for underwater habitats.

Thus, we can envisage a rebreather with an oxygen-supplementing gill to have a countercurrent exchanger. This would also have a hemoglobin-like oxygen transporter, which can then feed oxygenated liquid into a countercurrent exchange multiplier to provide the gaseous oxygen necessary to supplement the oxygen supply for the rebreather. Hemoglobin-like compounds could be modified to enhance oxygen loading and unloading on a chemical cue working in a similar way as the fish "Root effect" hemoglobins do within the fish countercurrent exchange multiplier. Or they could be designed to have a temperature-sensitive oxygen-carrying affinity.

It is through the maintenance of a concentration gradient that we get another biological mechanism that replaces liquid with gas. Nautilus and cuttlefish have gas-filled shell chambers that provide buoyancy control. Once the shell chamber has been formed, a wick-like porous structure uses osmosis to suck the liquid out of the chamber. As the pressure in the chamber drops, gas comes out of solution replacing the liquid (Chapter 5, Figures 5.4 and 5.5). However, it seems unlikely that this particular mechanism could provide the basis for oxygen supply to a diver, as the gas in the chamber is at a lower partial pressure than in the surrounding water. Also not all the gas is oxygen, and there is no obvious way to scale up this particular process to provide the oxygen levels needed by a diver. With some ingenuity it might be possible to mechanically create a pressure gradient that drives oxygen out of solution.

One way to do this would be to reduce the pressure in the surrounding water so that gas that includes oxygen comes out. Such a system is described in a 2007 U.S. Patent by Alon Bodner [23], which depicts a diver's vest containing two propellers that drive water through the vest and that, due to high tip speeds, introduce cavitation. This produces gas from the water that will contain dissolved air, which can be breathed by the diver.

The challenge thus far has not been to extract oxygen from water. This has been repeatedly demonstrated as a possibility. The real challenge is providing enough oxygen to satisfy the needs of humans, which is also human-driven. Artificial gills could also find use in other areas. Consider autonomous robots that harvest energy from local sources. Researchers at the Bristol Robotics Lab are developing robots that would digest food utilizing microbial fuel cells (MFCs). MFCs can require oxygen on the cathode side of the circuit. A far future scenario would have aquatic autonomous robots with gills: *Roboticus aquaticus*. They have looked at the use of a gill to provide the oxygen necessary for the cathode side, thus completing the circuit and receiving the electrons liberated during the microbial activity on the anode side of the battery cell [24].

There are substantial physiological challenges to making Cousteau's dream of *H. aquaticus* a reality: to have a new type of human with gills replacing lungs. It is clear from the discussion above that we can improve our ability to extract oxygen from seawater. Therefore, instead of redesigning the human we should consider augmenting the human with an artificial gill that collects oxygen from water and expels carbon dioxide to it. The challenge that we must face is how to do this reliably in a compact unit. Alan Bodner's device is compact but uses electric motors to separate oxygen from water using a cavitating propeller mechanism [23]. A passive gill that is driven by the muscles of our chest is still out of our reach. But with biomimetics, borrowing ideas from some of the examples listed above, we will find a way to do this. Our gill can be independent or could be used to supplement a device such as a rebreather. But if we must bring gas with us the ability to move vertically in the ocean is severely limited due to oxygen toxicity and the possibility of getting the bends when dissolved nitrogen leaves our body tissues. We could perhaps breathe a liquid such as a perfluorocarbon as discussed above. But this would require mechanical assistance.

Hence, for the moment, *Homo aquaticus* remains a dream, and we will continue to use our lungs to breathe air on SCUBA, but soon we could be using new devices that would feasibly supplement gas supply from water. After a day's work on the seabed we might also return to a submerged habitat that is independent of the surface with large-scale systems for gas exchange involving one or more of the ideas described above. The oxygen removed from the water could perhaps be stored chemically, rather than under pressure. Researchers at the University of Southern Denmark have recently developed a crystalline salt with a higher affinity for oxygen than myoglobin [25]; the oxygen storage agent within our muscles that in turn has a higher efficiency for oxygen than hemoglobin! There will be further advances enabling us to live in the sea, fulfilling Cousteau's vision.

References

1. Dugan, J. Portrait of *Homo aquaticus*, in *Edge of Awareness—25 Contemporary Essays*, R. Peck and N.E. Hoopes, Editors. 1967, New York, NY: Dell Publishing.
2. Ferretti, G. and Costa, M. Diversity in and adaptation to breath-hold diving in humans. *Comparative Biochemistry and Physiology Part A*: *Molecular & Integrative Physiology*, 2003. 136(1): 205–213.
3. DeLong, R.L. and Stewart, B.S. Diving patterns of northern elephant bull seals. *Marine Mammal Science*, 1991. 7(4): 369–384.
4. Watwood, S.L., Miller, P.J.O., Johnson, M., Madsen, P.T., and Tyack, P.L. Deep-diving foraging behaviour of sperm whales (*Physeter macrocephalus*). *Journal of Animal Ecology*, 2006. 75(3): 814–825.

5. Berta, A., Sumich, J.L., Kovacs, K.M., Folkens, P.A., and Adam, P.J. Respiration and diving physiology, in *Marine Mammals* (second edition). 2006, Burlington, MA: Academic Press. pp. 237–269.
6. Zimmer, W.M.X. and Tyack, P.L. Repetitive shallow dives pose decompression risk in deep-diving beaked whales. *Marine Mammal Science*, 2007. 23(4): 888–925.
7. Nieman, D.C., Trone, G.A., and Austin, M.D. A new handheld device for measuring resting metabolic rate and oxygen consumption. *Journal of the American Dietetic Association*, 2003. 103(5): 588–593.
8. Robb, W.L. Thin silicone membranes—Their permeation properties and some applications. *Annals of the New York Academy of Sciences*, 1968. 146(1): 119–137.
9. Cloud, W. Artificial gills: They'll let you breathe like a fish. *Popular Mechanics*, 1967. December: 69.
10. Ayres, W.A. Gill-Type Underwater Breathing Equipment and Methods for Reoxygenating Exhaled Breath. U.S. Patent Office. 1966. U.S. Patent #3,228,394.
11. Yang, M.-C. and Cussler, E.L. Artificial gills. *Journal of Membrane Science*, 1989. 42(3): 273–284.
12. Reiswig, H.M. The aquiferous systems of three marine demospongiae. *Journal of Morphology*, 1975. 145(4): 493–502.
13. Hentschel, U., Piel, J., Degnan, S.M., and Taylor, M.W. Genomic insights into the marine sponge microbiome. *Nature Reviews Microbiology*, 2012. 10(9): 641–654.
14. LaBarbera, M. and Vogel, S. The design of fluid transport systems in organisms. *American Scientist*, 1982. 70: 54–60.
15. Stucker, M., Struk, A., Altmeyer, P., Herde, M., Baumgartl, H., and Lubbers, D.W. The cutaneous uptake of atmospheric oxygen contributes significantly to the oxygen supply of human dermis and epidermis. *The Journal of Physiology*, 2002. 538(3): 985–994.
16. Fedder, M.E. and Burggren, W.W. Skin breathing in vertebrates. *Scientific American*, 1985. November: 126–142.
17. Heatwole, H. *Sea Snakes*. 1999, Sydney: UNSW Press. 148pp.
18. Shields, A.R., Fiser, B.L., Evans, B.A., Falvo, M.R., Washburn, S., and Superfine, R. Biomimetic cilia arrays generate simultaneous pumping and mixing regimes. *Proceedings of the National Academy of Science*, 2010. 107(36): 15670–15675.
19. den Toonder, J., Bos, F., Broer, R., Filippini, L., Gillies, M., de Goede, J., Mol, T. et al. Artifical cilia for active micro-fluidic mixing. *Lab on a Chip*, 2008. 8: 533–541.
20. Nagase, K.-I., Kohori, F., and Sakai, K. Development of a compact artificial gill using concentrated hemoglobin solution as the oxygen carrier. *Journal of Membrane Science*, 2003. 215(1–2): 281–292.
21. Nagase, K., Kohori, F., Sakai, K., and Nishide, H. Rearrangement of hollow fibers for enhancing oxygen transfer in an artificial gill using oxygen carrier solution. *Journal of Membrane Science*, 2005. 254(1–2): 207–217.
22. Kaisers, U., Kelly, K.P., and Busch, T. Liquid ventilation. *British Journal of Anaesthesia*, 2003. 91(1): 143–151.
23. Bodner, A. Open-Circuit Self-Contained Underwater Breathing Apparatus. U.S. Patent Office. 2007. U.S. Patent #7,278,422 B2.
24. Ieropoulos, I., Melhuish, C., and Greenman, J. Artificial gills for robots: MFC behaviour in water. *Bioinspiration & Biomimetics*, 2007. 2(3): S83.
25. Sundberg, J., Cameron, L.J., Southon, P.D., Kepert, C.J., and McKenzie, C.J. Oxygen chemisorption/desorption in a reversible single-crystal-to-single-crystal transformation. *ChemicalScience*, 2014. 5(10): 4017–4025.

Chapter 2 Swimming
through syrup

While snorkeling at the sea surface we naturally focus our eyes on distant objects: a rocky reef on the sea floor or a school of fish finding temporary shelter beneath our boat. But all around us in the water there are small creatures that are hunting food or avoiding predation. These include bacteria (about 1 μm long), single-celled dinoflagellate phytoplankton (10 μm to 1 mm diameter), crustaceans, fish (the smaller ones from 0.1 to 10 mm); some in their larval state that will soon seek a reef system to settle upon. Swimming is different for them: at minute lengths they experience water as a syrupy medium. Understanding how they swim at the submillimeter scale can provide insight into how we can revolutionize the design of microrobotic devices for swimming or pushing fluids.

Nineteenth century scientist Osborne Reynolds demonstrated how motion in fluids can be related to a dimensionless parameter that relates the relative influence of inertial forces to viscous forces [1]:

$$\text{Re} = \frac{LV\rho}{\eta} \tag{2.1}$$

His equation defines the Reynolds number (Re) where L is a characteristic length (e.g., diameter, fin length, etc.), ρ is the fluid density, η the viscosity, and V the velocity. The dimensionless Reynolds number, Re, provides a way to compare fluid flows across all length, velocity, density, and viscosity scales. For example, the Re* for a 2 m long scuba diver traveling at 0.5 m/s will be about 1 million (10^6). As the diver kicks there will be a transfer of momentum to the water, creating rotating masses of water, vortices, which will move backward as the diver moves forward.

The diver's forward motion is impeded by the fluid drag force,† proportional to the square of the velocity V. Thus for the diver, as velocity doubles, drag goes up by a factor of 4.

---

* The kinematic viscosity of water, $\upsilon \approx 10^{-6}$ m²/s was used for this calculation of the Reynolds number. Kinematic viscosity is viscosity η divided by density ρ.
† The drag force, F_D for instance, is the square of the velocity V multiplied by a reference area A, the fluid density ρ, and a coefficient of drag C_D (or lift C_L): $F_D = (1/2)C_D A\rho V^2$.

Bacteria, which is about 7 orders of magnitude shorter than a diver, inhabit a world in which viscous forces are dominant and the Re is substantially less than one (Figure 2.1) [2]. Although bacteria can swim fast for their size they cannot coast under their own inertia: when they stop swimming they stop moving. For example, the marine bacterium *Vibrio alginolyticus*, a source of infection and the

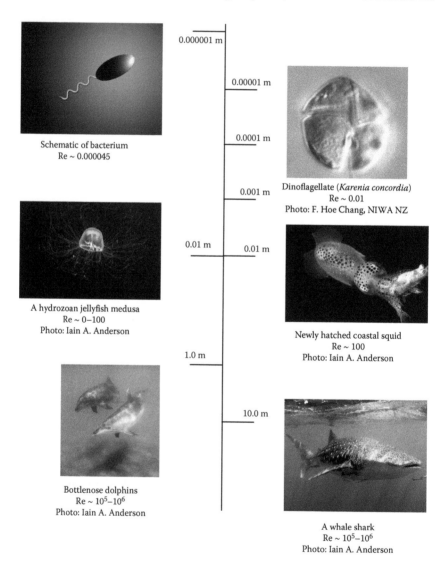

Schematic of bacterium
Re ~ 0.000045

0.000001 m

0.00001 m

0.0001 m

Dinoflagellate (*Karenia concordia*)
Re ~ 0.01
Photo: F. Hoe Chang, NIWA NZ

0.001 m

A hydrozoan jellyfish medusa
Re ~ 0–100
Photo: Iain A. Anderson

0.01 m

0.01 m

Newly hatched coastal squid
Re ~ 100
Photo: Iain A. Anderson

1.0 m

10.0 m

Bottlenose dolphins
Re ~ 10^5–10^6
Photo: Iain A. Anderson

A whale shark
Re ~ 10^5–10^6
Photo: Iain A. Anderson

Figure 2.1 Ocean organisms spanning 7 orders of magnitude in size with some Reynolds number (Re) data relative to the overall length.

lethal neurotoxin tetrodotoxin, "Zombie powder," which is present in the flesh of several species of pufferfish, can travel at 45 times its own length in a second. The Re for this bacterium is about 4.5×10^{-5}, 11 orders of magnitude smaller than the Re for the swimmer! Howard Berg of Harvard University [3] calculated the coasting distance for a fast swimming bacterium that he modeled as a simple sphere of radius 1 μm. His work indicated that when it stops swimming it will coast a distance that is less than the diameter of a hydrogen atom! The bacterium inhabits a world without inertia.

A key to swimming at low Re is to use nonreciprocating motion. Kicking a fin up and down is an example of a reciprocating motion: the upward stroke of the fin traces the same path as the downward stroke sending pockets of water backward. Do this at very low Re and you will not go anywhere. This point was raised by the Harvard University Nobel Laureate E.M. Purcell [4] who proposed a simple, 2 degrees-of-freedom microrobot that could swim when fully immersed at low Re (Figure 2.2) consisting of three rigid elements connected through two hinges, like a "boat with a rudder at each end." If one rudder moved up and down like the kicking of a fin (Figure 2.2a), the microrobot would wiggle sideways without any net motion away from where it sits; it would not swim. But if it moved its rudders in a nonreciprocal sequence (Figure 2.2b), then it would swim.

While following the basic principles for moving at low Re, it seems unlikely that Purcell's proposed microrobot would be able to navigate well. By this we mean steer in a controlled manner toward a destination. In contrast, bacteria can not only swim, they can also navigate toward food: they can steer.

We have been aware of bacterial motility from the eighteenth century when the inventor of the microscope, Antonie van Leeuwenhoek, first described the behavior of "clawed" animalcules that we now call microbes. In fact, 80% of bacteria [5] swim, but it was not clear until relatively recently how they did this. It was known that they moved using filamentous flagella and that at such low Re the forward thrust would be drag-based. Until the mid-1970s, biological opinion was divided on whether bacteria bent an active shape-changing flagellum in a wave-like manner or rotated a rigid flagellum like a propeller. Rotation would require a nanoscale rotary motor to do this. In 1973, a strong argument for the existence of such a motor was presented in a letter to *Nature* by Berg and Anderson [6]. By 1974, the rotation of the flagellum was clearly established in a clever experiment by Silverman and Simon [7], who used a mutant form of the bacterium *Escherichia coli* that was unable to produce a flagellum. When the mutant bacterium was attached to a microscope slide or another bacterium on its "hook," a sort of universal joint that links motor to flagellum (Figure 2.3), the bacterium would rotate. Their experiment, published in the journal *Nature*, clearly established that bacterial flagella are rotated by a motor, and this put an end to the "wave" hypothesis for bacterial swimming.

(a)

(b)

(1)

(2)

(3)

(4)

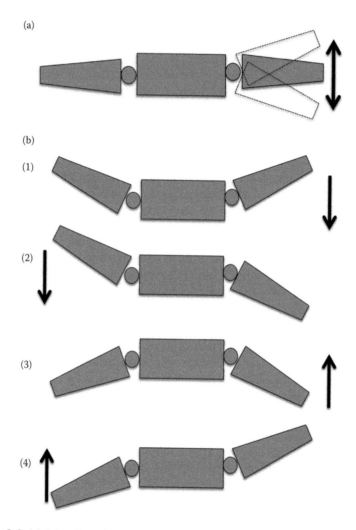

Figure 2.2 (a) A low Re swimming robot swimmer with two hinged fins, at left (L) and right (R) ends. In (a), only the right-hand side moves up and down. At very low Re there will be no movement away from where it sits. (b) Purcell demonstrated that if the robot moves its fins in a nonreciprocal pattern it will move from its position. An example of one nonreciprocal swimming pattern is shown: (1) RHS (right-hand side) clockwise, (2) LHS (left-hand side) counterclockwise, (3) RHS counterclockwise, and (4) LHS clockwise. (After Purcell, E.M. *American Journal of Physics*, 45(1), 3–11, 1977 [4].) (Drawings by Iain A. Anderson.)

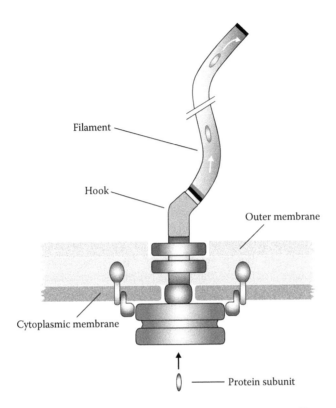

Figure 2.3 A schematic of the bacterial flagellum showing only the filament, hook, and the basal body, which anchors the device to the cell wall and includes the motor. This self-assembled protein complex is approximately 50 nm in diameter. The hook, between the filament and the motor acts like a universal joint. (From Macnab, R.M. *Journal of Bacteriology*, 181(23), 7149–7153, 1999 [8].) The flagellum is composed of 20 different proteins. The motor self-assembles in stages; built from smaller protein subunits in a process mediated by other proteins and described in a review article by Aizawa. (From Aizawa, S.-I. *Molecular Microbiology*, 19(1), 1–5, 1996 [5].) The primary rule for construction is the "sequential addition of simple components." For example, the external filament that can be several times the cell diameter in length is built using inside–out construction. The protein subunits are passed along its hollow interior to the end in the same way that a large chimney can be assembled brick by brick by masons working on the inside. (After Macnab, R.M. *Journal of Bacteriology*, 181(23), 7149–7153, 1999 [8]; Jarrell, K.F. and McBride, M.J. *Nature Reviews Microbiology*, 6, 466–476, 2008 [9].) (Redrawn by Mark T. Ryan.)

Unlike the substantially larger electric rotary inductive motors with which we are familiar, bacterial motors are driven by a flux of ions through the cell membrane that influence the rotor/stator protein junctions. The bacterial motor is a stepping motor in the sense that torque is generated using protein shape change (conformational change) during temporary attachment. These changes result in rotation of the helical flagellum; attached to the motor through the flexible hook.

It is better to use a helical flagellum than a typical propeller at low Re. At the center of a propeller is a hub that turns with the shaft and supports the blades (Figure 2.4). Turning a standard propeller at very low Re would still be expected to produce thrust. However, as one gets closer to the hub the circumferential speed of turning reduces with radius. Hence the hub region produces no thrust, but it does create drag and this is true at all values of Re. It follows that the best way to propel at very low Re is to reduce the area of the hub region and to have the propulsor surface as far away from the center as we can. We could perhaps introduce spokes to do this. But spokes would add a more drag-creating surface without contributing to propulsion. Making the lift-producing surface self-supporting,

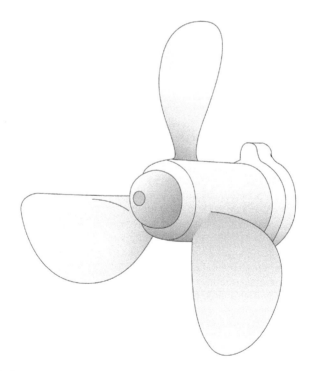

Figure 2.4 The screw propeller with its thrust-producing blades that are attached to a central hub; quite unlike the self-supporting helical filament of the bacterial flagellum (refer to Figure 2.3). (Drawing by Vivian L. Ward.)

through a continuous helix, like the bacterial flagellum (Figure 2.3), eliminates the need for drag-inducing spokes!

While a helical drive would be inappropriate for a motorboat it could potentially find use in other large-scale engineering applications. The wine bottle corkscrew that is slowly passing out of fashion with the advent of screw-top bottles is one practical example of a helical drive. Other applications, although not inspired by bacteria, include helical stirrers for mixing high-viscosity fluids such as cement or molasses! Such mixing machines have been around for over 100 years. A U.S. patent exists for a helical mixer for powdered or pulverized substances, which was awarded in 1909 [10]. A rotating helical structure can be used for propelling vehicles on sand, ice, and soil. For instance, the Soviet *ZIL-2906* was a large "screw-propelled vehicle" used for recovering cosmonauts from inaccessible terrain. Its body rested on two large cylinders, each surrounded with a helical flange. The screwing action of the turning cylinders drove the vehicle forward as it cut its own screw thread into the surface of the ground.

With its motorized flagellum the cell can now migrate to a place where nutrients are more abundant. For us, finding a destination is relatively easy given that we travel in two dimensions on roads with signposts and with global positioning systems and road signs to guide us. But bacteria occupy a three-dimensional world using cues that include chemical scent and magnetic field to guide them. To find "greener pastures" bacteria perform a biased random walk [3]; over time and with many changes of direction bacteria eventually find their way to a better place.

Bacterial motor control is limited to forward or reverse by changing the direction of rotation of the flagellum, clockwise or counterclockwise. And direction is linked to whether ions are moving into or out of the cell (H$^+$ for *E. coli* and Na$^+$ for *V. alginolyticus*). A positive gradient (higher ion density outside) that results in an inflow of ions past the motor produces a counterclockwise rotation of the flagellum when viewed from its rearward tip, resulting in a forward thrust. A negative ion gradient (higher ion density inside) results in a clockwise rotation of the flagellum and the ion gradient is controlled by the activity of ion pumps within the cell wall.

Thus, the cell can move forward and in reverse depending on the direction of rotation of the flagellum, but the flagellum is not actively steerable like the outboard motor to a boat. To travel on a different track requires a further application of forward/reverse motion anisotropy, as when we back a car into a parking space and then drive forward while rotating the steering wheel to draw the car toward the curb. In the place of a steering wheel, bacteria take advantage of changes in the attitude and orientation of flagella on reversal of the rotary motor. To understand how forward/reverse anisotropy can be realized consider two examples: For multiflagellar species such as *E. coli*, the two modes of locomotion are a counterclockwise "forward"-directed and a clockwise "reverse"-tumbling type [11]

(a)　　　　　　　　　　　　　　　　(b)

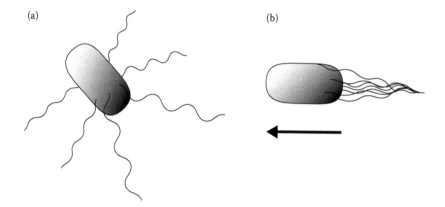

Figure 2.5 Clockwise rotation of the flagella results in tumbling (a). When all flagella are rotated counterclockwise, the flagella combine and the bacterium can propel itself forward (b). (After Egbert, M.D., Barandiaran, X.E., and Di Paolo, E.A. *PLoS Computational Biology*, 6(12), e1001004, 2010 [12].) (Drawing by Mark T. Ryan.)

(Figure 2.5). When moving forward, the counterclockwise rotation of the multiple flagella results in all the flagella becoming intertwined, which is facilitated through flexibility in their hooks so that they rotate as one and the motion is forward and directed. Reversal of one or more motors causes their flagella to separate from the bundle. The result is that the cell will cease to travel along one axis and will tumble. Reinstatement of counterclockwise rotation restores the intertwined union of flagella and the cell travels forward but in a different direction.

Species with a single flagellum, such as V. *alginolyticus*, can also use a "flick of the tail," to change direction [13] and this might involve a buckling instability in the flexible hook [14] (Figure 2.6). To move backward the helical tail turns clockwise and this pulls on the cell. But when the motor reverses so that the tail turns anticlockwise the cell is now pushed forward. This might cause the flexible hook between the relatively stiff tail and the cell to buckle as it is compressed and turned. But turning it could also stiffen the hook and this results in realignment of the tail so that it flicks, instigating a change in the swimming direction. Such a simple "turning by buckling" mechanism is simple and elegant and could be used for microrobotic applications.

Whether through reverse tumbling or flicking its tail, the bacterium can head off on a new course, using chemical or magnetic cues to identify a promising direction and then bias its random "walk" (e.g., time spent running forward or reverse/tumbling) so that it can navigate to a goal of some sort. "Navigation" also requires something akin to memory [15] for the cell needs to compare present and past sensory data, in this case a chemical concentration; quite a remarkable feat for an organism that is order of 1 μm long.

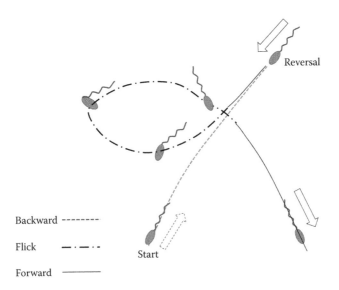

Figure 2.6 Schematic illustrating the sequence of the tail-flicking mechanism of *V. alginolyticus*. Start: Backward swimming followed by motor reversal so that it swims forward. The instability associated with the tail now leads to the tail-flicking motion. The trail realigns its axis with the bacterium that now swims forward in a new direction. (Adapted from Xie, L. et al. *Proceedings of the National Academy of Sciences*, 108(6), 2246–2251, 2011 [13].) (Drawing by Iain A. Anderson.)

Evidence suggests that the efficiency of the bacterial motor is quite low. In an article published posthumously, titled "Efficiency of propulsion by a rotating flagellum," E.M. Purcell evaluated the effectiveness of any flagellum-like propulsor operating at very low Re [16]. He performed an ingenious experiment, dropping models of flagella (simple wire helices) through a viscous fluid (he used silicone oil). He measured the speed at which the models sank through the fluid, and their rotation. In a second experiment, he dropped models made of two helices of opposite handedness, joined end to end, through the oil. These models did not rotate because their rotatory torques canceled each other out. He repeated both experiments using helices with various pitch angles and lengths, and calculated their efficiency; defined as the work required to pull a cell through the water divided by the work by the "man inside turning the crank," which rotates the flagellum. The calculated efficiencies were all less than 1%. This is within the ballpark of efficiency data presented by Stephen Childress [17] of New York University; about 3% for a helical flagellum.

Why does the bacterial cell use a propulsor to seek food if the propulsion is so inefficient? Purcell went on to show that even at this low efficiency the power required would be rather small, about 0.5 W/kg, when compared with its energy budget, hence it was like "driving a Datsun in Saudi Arabia." It probably does not really matter much to the cell how efficient the motor/flagellum is; what does matter is that it gives the bacterium an affordable advantage to collect nutrients compared with just sitting and waiting for diffusion to deliver nutrients.

The ability to get around at the micrometer scale autonomously without the need to recharge the battery has inspired some novel ideas for nanorobots, which combine living actuators with engineered objects. For example, Martel and coworkers [18] have groomed magnetotactic bacteria to act as robots for transporting drugs within the body. These bacteria are sensitive to magnetic fields, containing membrane-bound nanoparticles of magnetite. Although these cells are influenced by other sensory cues, they persistently swim along lines of force of a magnetic field. They can be encouraged to swim in a man-made magnetic field provided that the field exceeds the strength of the Earth's own field. Thus, they can perform the role of drug mules within the body by delivering drugs and potentially be detectable on MRI (magnetic resonance imaging) so that their location can be tracked. Martel et al. have proposed several ways for packaging and moving drugs inside the body by means of several thousand attached magnetotactic bacteria. Angelani and Leonardo [19] suggested making a living nanorobot that would use teams of bacteria. The basic idea was to immerse objects in a field of bacteria and allow the bacteria to cluster on the objects in such a way that they push them in a preferred direction.

The flagellum need not be a rigid corkscrew. For instance, sperm use an active flagellum that is a flexible shape-changing molecular motor driven in much the same way as a cilium, with individual actuators (dynein molecules) acting on rods (made from microtubules) extending inside the length of the flagellum. These flagella can transmit waves along their length and also mimic the motion of the bacterial flagellum. The flagellum of sea urchin sperm [20] typically produces 1.5 wavelengths beating in a sinusoidal manner and has been seen to swim using planar or helical waves in its flagellum [21].

Bacteria migrate toward a goal by a biased random walk but sperm and other swimming microorganisms can steer toward their target. They follow a helical path, as though they were swimming alongside an imaginary screw thread; like a rocket with a faulty guidance system. But their guidance is not faulty. In fact, helical swimming is a reliable and effective way of homing in on a target and does not require fine-tuning [22]. The target could be a food source or, in the case of the sea urchin sperm, an unfertilized sea urchin egg.

The homing mechanism is formally known as a *helical klinotaxis*. The phenomenon was reported over 100 years ago in an article by Jennings [23], who described how the same side of the organism's body is always directed to the inside of the helix. He offered an explanation for this: that helical swimming provides a way for an organism, "no matter how misshapen and irregular" to follow a course "which is, in effect, equivalent to a straight line." This argument is weakened by the observation that other creatures with symmetric body plans swim this way, such as larval sea squirts (ascidians) that perform helical klinotaxis through controlled curvature of the tail [24]. These creatures are a few millimeters long and swim from several minutes to 10 days in the plankton before attaching themselves to a surface and growing into tube-like structures attached to the seabed.

Dinoflagellates (Figure 2.1), members of the phytoplankton (they are plants), whose name is based on the Greek word "dinos" (whirling) [25], beat the water with two whip-like flagella. A trailing flagellum pushes it forward that, due to its asymmetric position, causes the cell to rotate. The other flagellum lies in a groove around the body that also rotates the cell [26]. The cell can use these two flagella to control the direction of its helical path, by adjusting the ratio of the spin frequencies about two axes: longitudinal and transverse. The vector sum of these two angular velocities determines the axis of the helix [26].

Sensitive algae that also swim along a helical path can steer so that they orient relative to a light source [27]. These algae have a light-sensitive spot that is less than 50 wavelengths of light across. The spot detects a periodic change in light intensity as the algal cell rotates, and its signal is used for orientation of the swimming direction. Examples of helical klinotaxis like these provide inspiration for microrobots that can track using a single sensor [28] (Figure 2.7); and have been demonstrated in both aquatic and terrestrial robots that can detect a light intensity gradient, and navigate up the gradient [29].

If the wave-like motion of flagella can drive a propulsor, the same mechanism can be used as a pump. We could, for instance, anchor a flagellum thus stopping it from moving and in doing this create a mechanism for transporting fluid. Now imagine a vast array of flagella working in unison and all pumping into the same cavity so that they produce a net flow of water. This describes the sponge with its internal chambers lined with choanocytes, each of which waves a single flagellum (see Figure 1.3, Chapter 1). The flow of water created by a flagellum enables the entrapment of food within microvilli at the base of each choanocyte. The sum of all flagella beating water produces a net flow through the sponge and is vented. Imagine an array of choanocyte-like microactuators that could transport fluid across a membrane, promoting gas diffusion within an artificial gill, for instance, as discussed in Chapter 1.

For low Re fluid transport, the cilia array is center stage. Cilia utilize the same microtubular molecular motor as sperm flagellum but are typically much shorter, in the order of 10 μm long. The kinematics of ciliary beating is nonreciprocating: the cilium performs a power stroke, like a swinging baseball bat followed by a low-profile curved recovery stroke (Figure 2.8). Individual cilia enable the swimming of ciliates and other microbes, but when aligned in large-scale arrays they work together to transport fluid across millimeter scale surfaces. Examples

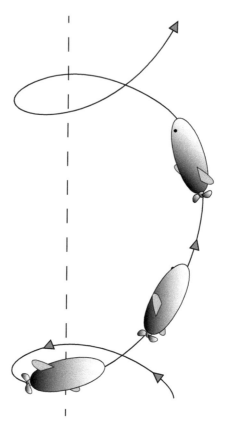

Figure 2.7 Hypothetical helical klinotaxis microrobot driven by a single, small steerable propeller. It follows a helical path guided by its single light or chemical sensor. (Drawing by Mark T. Ryan.)

include the movement of water through the mussel and the transport of mucus along the wall of our trachea. Like the Mexican wave produced by a crowd at a football match, arrays of cilia generate a pattern of actuation that is referred to as a metachronal wave.

Cilia arrays can drive relatively large organisms, tens of centimeters long: the ctenophores or comb jellies (Figure 2.9).

These fragile creatures require full immersion in water to support their soft bodies. If touched by hand or flipper the ctenophore's body will be damaged. But despite their fragility they are an evolutionary success story, with a fossil record of half a billion years or more. They have no brain but react to sensory information from water and gravity [30]. Some species that grow to a dozen or more centimeters are frequently encountered near the surface of the sea; drawing attention

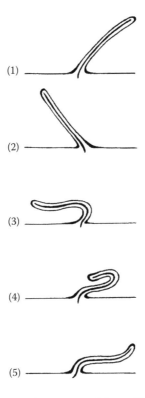

(1)

(2)

(3)

(4)

(5)

Figure 2.8 When a cilium beats, its movement is qualitatively similar to a swimmer's arm doing the breaststroke. There is a fast power stroke (1 and 2) that pushes fluid backward. This is followed by a recovery stroke (3–5). (Drawing by Annelise Wiebkin.)

to themselves as their cilia comb swimming paddles stroke the water, producing a colorful light display from refracted sunlight.

The cilia plate paddles are each composed of thousands of extra long cilia, arranged in eight rows longitudinally from the mouth to the rear end. In some species, the plates can be up to 2 mm wide and 50 µm thick [31] and up to 2 mm long [32], with cilia packed together like bristles of a house-painter's brush. When triggered, the cilia within each plate move in unison, operating at Re of the order of 100 [31]. During swimming, the plates also move one after the other, in a wave of actuation. Each plate is triggered by the one behind it, producing a wave of actuation that moves along the row from the rear toward the front of the animal [32,33]. When triggered, a plate pushes water in a power stroke followed by a soft spaghetti-like recoil; resembling the movement of the single cilium depicted in Figure 2.8.

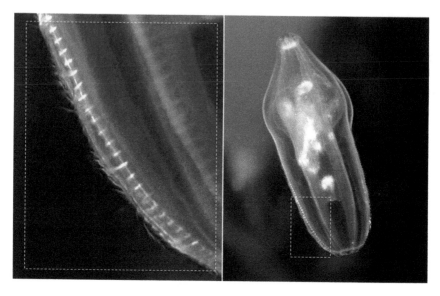

Figure 2.9 A comb jellyfish (ctenophore) in the Poor Knights Islands (New Zealand). The mouth is at the top of the image; this is the direction the animal swims. The magnified portion of the image depicts two waves of cilia comb plate activation. Each plate contains thousands of extra long cilia that move in unison when triggered. (Photo by Iain A. Anderson.)

The collective action of multiple waves along the eight rows produces a net thrust that drives the ctenophore forward. Using several ctenophore species as his experimental subjects, Sydney Tamm, at Indiana University's Department of Zoology, showed that in some species prevention of plate movement (by holding it down for instance) can stop the wave from continuing along the row, whereas in others (lobate type) the wave would proceed indicating that neural pathways for plate triggering might exist [33]. This metachronal movement is common to all animals that have close-packed limbs who would trip over one another if they did not move in a coordinated manner. This can be seen in other sea creatures such as brine shrimp (*Artemia*) and in land animals such as millipedes.

The control strategy has some clear advantages: each comb plate acts directly, eliminating the need for complex transmission systems, and a plate responds only when influenced by its neighbor either mechanically or neurally. This simple control strategy has been mimicked using electronic artificial muscle technology based on the dielectric elastomer [34]. Researchers at the University of Auckland's Biomimetics Lab have developed demonstration conveyor devices inspired by the ctenophore comb row [35]. The conveyor is composed of an array

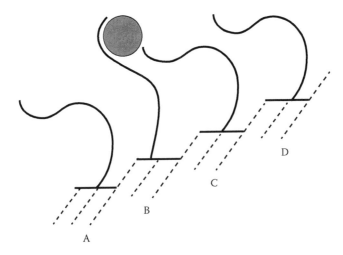

Figure 2.10 An array of touch-sensitive actuators. The actuator at B pushes an object forward to C. The actuator at C is touch sensitive and when triggered, will push the object further forward. (After O'Brien, B.M. Simulation, *Fabrication, and Control of Biomimetic Actuator Arrays*, 2010. Auckland Bioengineering Institute, The University of Auckland, Auckland [36].) (Drawing by Mark T. Ryan.)

of paddles driven by artificial muscle actuators. Each individual touch-sensitive actuator works on a very simple control rule: turn on and push the object further forward when touched by the preceding actuator (Figure 2.10).

Arrays of microactuators that mimic the motion depicted in Figure 2.8 can also provide microfluidic pumping and mixing in lab-on-a-chip devices. Researchers at Philips [37] have produced electrostatically actuated curled microbeams that are double layer: consisting of a polymer (1 µm thick) with a much thinner chromium conductor bonded to it. Electric charge causes the curled beam to extend and the extension and relaxation of the beam arrays pumps the fluid. These arrays can then be printed onto a lab-on-a-chip for closely controlled fluid transport and mixing. Another system consists of a magnetically activated array of 700 nm thick and 25 µm high cilia composed of flexible magnetic nanoparticles that are dispersed in silicone [38,39]. When the magnetic field is turned on, the cilia align with the field, and so switching the field can be used to drive the whole array for pumping and mixing fluids at the micron scale.

Our examples have, thus far, provided natural solutions for propulsion and pumping at low Re. Among the many challenges for microrobotics is chemical sensing as this relates to homing in on a target that might involve, say, a site of drug delivery to an organ. One might wish to develop a microrobot with a sensory device that enables it to taste the fluid within which it is moving. We have discussed the homing technique of helical klinotaxis. Alternatively, the ability to sense chemicals could be useful in a stationary device, part of a lab-on-a-chip technology. So, how can we get the microdevice to taste the water when the boundary layer is quite thick, as one would expect for a low Re flow? Nature provides a solution that is associated with the judicious use of "hairs" and bristles. For some planktonic crustaceans leg hair is a real asset for swimming, chemical sensing and intercepting planktonic food. Small crustaceans such as copepods use bristles (setae) for swimming and for filtering water for food (Figure 2.11) [40]. They can also collect water for chemical sampling. Their swimming appendages are multifunctional and this ability is based on a transition in Re.

The appendages of some small crustacea are used not only as paddles for swimming but also as sieves for filter-feeding. But a paddle must present a solid surface while a filter has holes in it. How can this paradox be resolved? Swimming appendages with setae, when operated at very low Re of 0.1 or less, perform like paddles. The boundary layer across each seta is of comparable thickness to the gaps between them. But the same seta-bearing appendages operating at much higher Re, a flow regime where boundary layers are less than the inter-setal spacing, become sieves [40,41].

Thus, for setae of appropriate size and spacing there might exist a transition zone that could be exploited by the organism in swimming, feeding, and chemical sensing. Sweeping a bristly sieve next to an edge, or coordinated sweeping between adjacent appendages could affect whether the bristly appendage acts like a paddle or sieve. If the Reynolds number is too low then changes in velocity are unlikely to influence the "leakiness" of the appendage; that will remain paddle-like. Swinging at a higher velocity might alter performance from being paddle-like to sieve-like.

Setae for copepods, krill, and other small crustaceans operate across a broad range of Re from 10^{-4} to 1 (see the review in Cheer and Koehl [41]). Koehl has suggested that for closely spaced setae, the Re number at which transition might occur is on the order of 1 [42]. Thus, a strategy for chemical sensing, used by crustaceans, is to flick a sensory appendage such as an antennule fast in one direction so that fresh fluid moves through and past setae for sample collection, followed by a slow, low Re number recovery stroke in which no new fluid is collected [42]. To the best of our knowledge this has not been achieved in a lab-on-a-chip device but could be a worthwhile goal for a chemical sensor.

It is clear that copepod crustaceans and the vast myriad of other small micron and millimeter scale creatures, that live and move round in the plankton at low Re, are easy to overlook. However, we should pay attention to how they move about and control water as they can inform us on the design of new devices that can move, navigate, pump, and mix at low Re when water is like syrup.

(a)

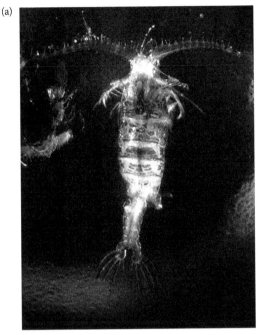

(b)

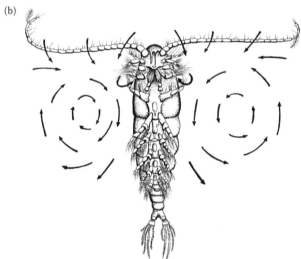

Figure 2.11 (a) A copepod that is approximately 2 mm long caught in a plankton trawl. Copepod limbs are used for both swimming and feeding. (b) The feeding limbs beat very fast, about 50 Hz and this sets up water currents (vortices) that bring food particles to their setae. (Photo by Dr. Steve O'Shea. Drawing by Annelise Wiebkin.)

35

References

1. Reynolds, O. An experimental investigation of the circumstances which determine whether the motion of water shall be direct or sinuous, and of the law of resistance in parallel channels. *Proceedings of the Royal Society of London Series B*, 1883. 35: 84–89.
2. Englert, D.L., Jayaraman, A., and Manson, M.D. Microfluidic techniques for the analysis of bacterial chemotaxis, in *CHEMOTAXIS Methods in Molecular Biology*. J. Jin and D. Hereld, Editors. 2009, New York, NY: Humana Press, Springer. pp. 1–23.
3. Berg, H.C. *Random Walks in Biology*. 1983, Princeton, NJ: Princeton University Press.
4. Purcell, E.M. Life at low Reynold's number. *American Journal of Physics*, 1977. 45(1): 3–11.
5. Aizawa, S.-I. Flagellar assembly in *Salmonella typhimurium*. *Molecular Microbiology*, 1996. 19(1): 1–5.
6. Berg, H.C. and Anderson, R.A. Bacteria swim by rotating their flagellar filaments. *Nature*, 1974. 245: 380–382.
7. Silverman, M. and Simon, M. Flagellar rotation and the mechanism of bacterial motility. *Nature*, 1974. 249: 73–74.
8. Macnab, R.M. The bacterial flagellum: Reversible rotary propeller and type III export apparatus. *Journal of Bacteriology*, 1999. 181(23): 7149–7153.
9. Jarrell, K.F. and McBride, M.J. The surprisingly diverse ways that prokaryotes move. *Nature Reviews Microbiology*, 2008. 6: 466–476.
10. Gedge, J.F., Editor. Sifting and Mixing Machine. January 15, 1909. U.S. Patent Office. U.S. Patent #934603 A.
11. Manson, M.D., Armitage, J.P., Hoch, J.A., and Macnab, R.M. Bacterial locomotion and signal transduction. *Journal of Bacteriology*, 1998. 180(5): 1009–1022.
12. Egbert, M.D., Barandiaran, X.E., and Di Paolo, E.A. A minimal model of metabolism-based chemotaxis. *PLoS Computational Biology*, 2010. 6(12): e1001004.
13. Xie, L., Altindal, T., Chattopadhyay, S., and Wu, X.-L. Bacterial flagellum as a propeller and as a rudder for efficient chemotaxis. *Proceedings of the National Academy of Sciences*, 2011. 108(6): 2246–2251.
14. Son, K., Guasto, J.S., and Stocker, R. Bacteria can exploit a flagellar buckling instability to change direction. *Nature Physics*, 2013. 9(8): 494–498.
15. Macnab, R.M. and Koshland, D.E. The gradient-sensing mechanism in bacterial chemotaxis. *Proceedings of the National Academy of Sciences*, 1972. 69(9): 2509–2512.
16. Purcell, E.M. The efficiency of propulsion by a rotating flagellum. *Proceedings of the National Academy of Sciences*, 1997. 94: 11307–11311.
17. Childress, S. *Mechanics of Swimming and Flying*. 1977: Courant Institute of Mathematical Sciences, New York, NY: New York University.
18. Martel, S., Mohammadi, M., Felfoul, O., Lu, Z., and Pouponneau, P. Flagellated magnetotactic bacteria as controlled MRI-trackable propulsion and steering systems for medical nanorobots operating in the human microvasculature. *International Journal of Robotics Research*, 2009. 28(4): 571–582.
19. Angelani, L. and Leonardo, R.D. Geometrically biased random walks in bacteria-driven micro-shuttles. *New Journal of Physics*, 2010. 12(11): 113017.
20. Rikmenspoel, R. Movement of sea urchin sperm flagella. *Journal of Cell Biology*, 1978. 76(2): 310–322.
21. Woolley, D.M. and Vernon, G.G. A study of helical and planar waves on sea urchin sperm flagella, with a theory of how they are generated. *Journal of Experimental Biology*, 2001. 204(7): 1333–1345.
22. Friedrich, B.M. and Jülicher, F. Chemotaxis of sperm cells. *Proceedings of the National Academy of Sciences*, 2007. 104(33): 13256–13261.

23. Jennings, H.S. On the significance of the spiral swimming of organisms. *American Naturalist*, 1901. 35(413): 369–378.
24. McHenry, M.J. Mechanisms of helical swimming: Asymmetries in the morphology, movement and mechanics of larvae of the ascidian *Distaplia occidentalis*. *Journal of Experimental Biology*, 2001. 204(17): 2959–2973.
25. Spector, D.L. Dinoflagellates: An introduction, in *Dinoflagellates*, D.L. Spector, Editor. 1984, Orlando, FL: Academic Press Ltd.
26. Fenchel, T. How dinoflagellates swim. *Protist*, 2001. 152(4): 329–338.
27. Foster, K.W. and Smyth, R.D. Light antennas in phototactic algae. *Microbiological Reviews*, 1980. 44(4): 572–630.
28. Pell, C.A., Crenshaw, H.C., Janet, J., and Kemp, M. Devices and Methods for Orienting and Steering in Three-Dimensional Space. August 10, 1999. U.S. Patent #6378801 B1.
29. Long, J.H.J., Lammert, A.C., Pell, C.A., Kemp, M., Strother, J.A., Crenshaw, H.C., and McHenry, M.J. A navigational primitive: Biorobotic implementation of cycloptic helical klinotaxis in planar motion. *Journal of Oceanic Engineering*, 2011. 29(29): 795–806.
30. Chiel, H.J. and Beer, R.D. The brain has a body: Adaptive behavior emerges from interactions of nervous system, body and environment. *Trends in Neurosciences*, 1997. 20(12): 553–557.
31. Matsumoto, G.I. Swimming movements of ctenophores, and the mechanics of propulsion by ctene rows. *Hydrobiologia*, 1991. 216–217(1): 319–325.
32. Wiederhold, M.L. Mechanosensory transduction in "Sensory" and "Motile" cilia. *Annual Review of Biophysics and Bioengineering*, 1976. 5(1): 39–62.
33. Tamm, S.L. Mechanisms of ciliary co-ordination in ctenophores. *Journal of Experimental Biology*, 1973. 59(1): 231–245.
34. Anderson, I.A., Gisby, T.A., McKay, T.G., O'Brien, B.M., and Calius, E.P. Multi-functional dielectric elastomer artificial muscles for soft and smart machines. *Journal of Applied Physics*, 2012. 112(4): 041101.
35. O'Brien, B., Gisby, T., Calius, E., Xie, S., and Anderson, I. FEA of dielectric elastomer minimum energy structures as a tool for biomimetic design. *Proceedings of SPIE*, 2009. 7287: 728706–1.
36. O'Brien, B.M. *Simulation, Fabrication, and Control of Biomimetic Actuator Arrays*, 2010. Auckland Bioengineering Institute, The University of Auckland, Auckland.
37. den Toonder, J., Bos, F., Broer, R., Filippini, L., Gillies, M., de Goede, J., Mol, T. et al. Artificial cilia for active micro-fluidic mixing. *Lab on a Chip*, 2008. 8: 533–541.
38. Shields, A.R., Fiser, B.L., Evans, B.A., Falvo, M.R., Washburn, S., and Superfine, R. Biomimetic cilia arrays generate simultaneous pumping and mixing regimes. *Proceedings of the National Academy of Science*, 2010. 107(36): 15670–15675.
39. Khaderi, S.N., Craus, C.B., Hussong, J., Schorr, N., Belardi, J., Westerweel, J., Prucker, O., Ruhe, J., den Toonder, J.M.J., and Onck, P.R. Magnetically actuated artificial cilia for microfluidic propulsion. *Lab on a Chip*, 2011. 11(12): 2002–2010.
40. Koehl, M.A.R. and Strickler, J.R. Copepod feeding currents: Food capture at low Reynolds number. *Limnology and Oceanography*, 1981. 26(6): 1062–1073.
41. Cheer, A.Y.L. and Koehl, M.A.R. Paddles and rakes: Fluid flow through bristled appendages of small organisms. *Journal of Theoretical Biology*, 1987. 129(1): 17–39.
42. Koehl, M.A.R. The fluid mechanics of arthropod sniffing in turbulent odor plumes. *Chemical Senses*, 2006. 31(2): 93–105.

Chapter 3 The hydrostat

Ocean organisms that lack a rigid skeleton provide inspiration for the design of soft and extensible robots capable of changing shape, stretching out, reaching around corners, and manipulating objects. The octopus, for instance, can dexterously move and arrange rocks and shells, and change its shape for streamlined swimming (Figure 3.1). Anemones can assume a cylindrical form and stand tall or contract to small round jelly-like blobs only a fraction of their full height (Figure 3.2). All are hydrostats, using the near incompressibility of water (or water-saturated tissue) to change shape, stiffness, and provide a rigid skeleton-like support for muscle.

Water's incompressibility can be illustrated in the following thought experiment: imagine filling two balloons, one with air and one with an equal volume of water. After filling and sealing we transport both from the ocean surface to the deck of the *Titanic* at approximately 3.8 km depth. To calculate their respective volumes at depth we can use compressibility data for water [1], for the water-filled balloon, and Boyle's Law for the air-filled balloon. Boyle's Law states that gas volume will be inversely proportional to pressure at fixed temperature. Here, we make the simplifying assumption that the temperature at depth is the same as the surface temperature. At such a high pressure, of over 370 atmospheres, the balloon filled with air would occupy less than 0.3% of its original volume at the surface, whereas the balloon filled with water would look much the same occupying 98% of its sea level volume. This near incompressibility is at the core of the hydrostat mechanism.

Perhaps, the most commonly encountered living hydrostats are the sea anemones. They can make themselves stiff or flaccid and, through actuation of muscle groups, can tip over to one side or the other and manipulate captured prey toward the mouth. Some species can retract their tentacles and deflate their bodies to become a small oblate bump on a rock, or they can inflate to a tall cylinder many times the deflated volume with pumped-up tentacles (Figure 3.2). They are relatives of (cnidarian) jellyfish and so are also similar in body plan: two layers of cells, one on the outside and one lining the gut confine a jelly-like substance, mesoglea, in between. Sea anemones pump water internally through two ciliated channels (siphonoglyphs) at opposite sides of the mouth or pharynx. As water enters the body the volume increases. With the mouth closed, an anemone can maintain constant volume. Muscle groups that are arranged around the circumference can contract and make the anemone tall and slender. Contraction of muscles that run longitudinally up and down the body can make the anemone short and fat.

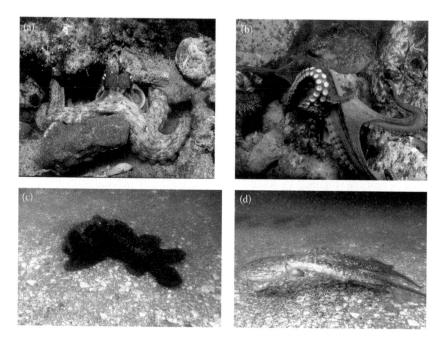

Figure 3.1 (a) An octopus manipulates a large rock. This one attacked the photographer's camera reaching out and wrapping one of its arms firmly around the firing cord that runs between the camera and the strobe light. (b) This octopus is making an aggressive display. (c) An octopus over sand in the shallows near a beach on New Zealand's Coromandel Peninsula. (d) The octopus depicted in (c) changed color and pattern, lengthened its body to assume a streamlined pose and jetted away. (Photos by Iain A. Anderson.)

The shape assumed by the anemone is largely due to mesoglea; a composite material that is sandwiched between the cell-lined walls, mostly composed of collagen fibers in a watery gel. As water goes into the anemone the mesoglea responds by slowly stretching. This is reminiscent of the slow change in shape under pressure of viscous solids such as modeling clay and builder's putty. But clay or putty will hold their shape when the pressure of the hand is removed. The mesoglea of the anemone is different to this for if the anemone were to pump water out it would eventually shrink back to its original size. This is a characteristic of an elastic material. The mesoglea is viscoelastic, displaying characteristics that are both elastic and viscous.

The force required to stretch a viscoelastic material in a test machine will also depend on the rate of stretch. A slow rate of stretch will require less force than a fast one. And if the tension is removed the viscoelastic material will slowly creep back to its original shape.

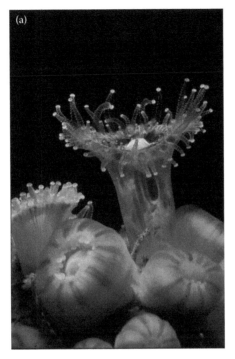

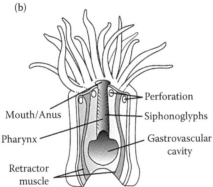

Figure 3.2 (a) A single jewel anemone (*Actinia tenebrosa*) in New Zealand's Poor Knights Islands presents a tall cylindrical body. Surrounding anemones of the same species were touched by the photographer's finger causing them to retract their tentacles and close down and assume a round shape. (Photo by Iain A. Anderson.) (b) While expanding, water is slowly pumped into the anemone under the action of cilia arrays (siphonoglyphs) that line two opposing ends of the pharynx. The pharynx acts like a nonreturn valve that can also be opened to receive food into the gastrovascular cavity and to release internal water when the anemone is reducing in size under muscle action. (Drawing by Vivian L. Ward.)

Mesoglea is less compliant circumferentially than longitudinally [2]. Its material properties are direction-dependent due to orientation of collagen fibers [2]. The anemone is a fiber-reinforced hydrostat. So, when the anemone slowly fills with water the pressure causes the body wall to stretch. Collagen fibers will slide past each other but many of these fibers are also oriented parallel to the major stress axes of the body, so that the inflated anemone assumes a cylindrical shape instead of a spherical one. Very large strains are possible (over 300%), with very low power expenditure due to the slow rate of filling. Additionally, the collagen fibers in the outer layers of the mesoglea are organized in a crossed-helical array, rather like a mesh stocking.

Although useful for slow-directed shape change, the anemone mesoglea mechanism would not be practical in a fast robotic manipulator on a car assembly line. There are many living examples of relatively "fast" hydrostat mechanisms that employ stiff windings of collagen around the outside of the body [3] for longitudinal extensions, contractions, and controlled stiffening under the influence of living muscle. Nemertean worms also known as ribbon worms, for instance, have stiff collagen fibers in their skin that are joined together to form inextensible helical cords and the helical arrangement allows some species to extend over 6 times their "shortened" length [4]. This also renders them resistant to twisting [5].

Consider a segment of a worm-like body modeled as a cylindrical elastic structure that is filled with water and wrapped around the outside with inextensible cords arranged as left- and right-handed helices (Figure 3.3). The angle that the mesh makes with the longitudinal direction will determine how the structure responds to further filling: it can be shown that a high mesh angle of, for instance, 85° will result in expansion and a low mesh angle of, say, 17° will cause it to contract [4].

For nemertean worms, at least, there is no external pump supplying water to the body. A relatively constant volume and the stiffness of the collagen fibers set limits on how far it can extend or shorten its body under muscle control.

McKibben actuators (Figure 3.4) used in robotics [6] combine a rubber cylinder supported within a stiff braided mesh. They contract when fluid is added. While the McKibben actuator can be lightweight and portable it usually requires the regulated delivery of high-pressure air or water from a relatively large and heavy pump, compressor, or gas cylinder, although there is growing interest in using water or oil instead of air as such hydraulic muscles can work faster [7] and perform as hydrostats.

The skin of sharks is almost entirely composed of a crossed-helical collagen array, oriented between 50° and 70° between pectoral and anal fins (Figure 3.5). This can be used to impart stiffness to the skin that provides anchoring for the

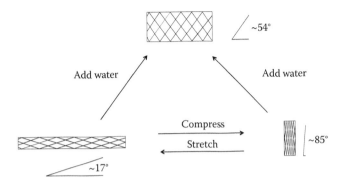

Figure 3.3 A segment of a hose (or worm) with an external inextensible braid. On the left it is stretched. The segment will resist further stretching when the inextensible cords become taut. We have them starting from the arbitrary angle of 17°. If it were forcibly shortened by longitudinal muscle action at a constant volume it will eventually assume the profile on the right, with a high cord angle; in this example 85°. In between the two positions the cross-sectional shape will not be round, assuming an elliptical shape, for instance. Adding water to the extended hose (or worm) on the left-hand side will result in contraction. For the contracted segment on the right, adding water will result in expansion. At maximum volume the angle is approximately 54°. (Drawing by Iain A. Anderson.)

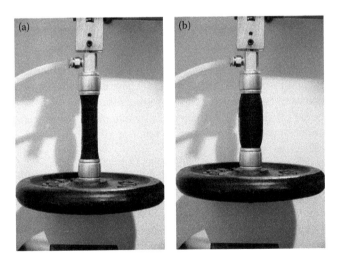

Figure 3.4 (a) A Festo fluidic artificial muscle that consists of a rubber cylinder supported within a braided metal mesh. In (b), the pressurized muscle lifting a 5 kg weight. (Photos by Allan Veale.)

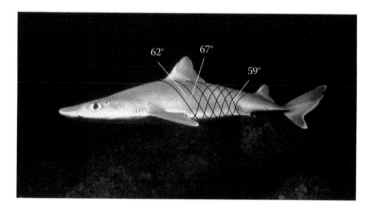

Figure 3.5 A school shark also known by the rather unfortunate name of soupfin shark (*Galeorhinus galeus*) in the Poor Knights Islands, New Zealand. Typical collagen angles are indicated. Note the heterocercal tail in which the top part is longer than the bottom. This tail sends water backward and down creating lift at the rear of the shark's body. (After Wainwright, S.A., Vosburgh, F., and Hebrank, J.H. *Science*, 202(4369), 747–749, 1978 [8].) (Photo by Iain A. Anderson.)

swimming muscles; there is strong evidence that the stiffening effected by the collagen plays a central role in swimming [8]. Measurements of pressure beneath the skin of a lemon shark showed an almost 10-fold rise between rest and bursts of fast swimming. Such pressure increases can lead to substantial rises in surface skin stiffness [8]. The collagen fibers also extend out to the tail fin so that the body muscles directly pull the tail fin left and right during swimming.

We could emulate muscle using electroactive polymer artificial muscles based on the dielectric elastomer [9,10]. Such "muscles" have already been used to control the deformations of an air-inflated rubber rolling robot [11] and an air-swimming fish-like blimp [12] (Figure 7.9, Chapter 7). It remains for engineers to explore the use of an incompressible fluid such as water or oil in the place of air within a hollow electroactive polymer.

Now imagine a hydraulic system that uses muscles arranged in multiple orientations to effect shape change (Figure 3.6).

The starfish tube foot is such an actuator. Starfish that occupy all seafloor habitats from rocky outcrops to loose sand, march from place to place on arms that support hundreds of hydrostat tube feet that are actuated both hydraulically and by muscle (Figure 3.7). Some species use their feet to excavate the sand beneath them so that they appear to sink beneath the surface of the sand, where they can hide in ambush: a star-shaped outline on the sand with only the light-sensitive organs on the tips of their arms exposed, betrays their presence. These sand stars have tube feet that are pointed, like the bottom ends of ancient Roman amphorae,

44

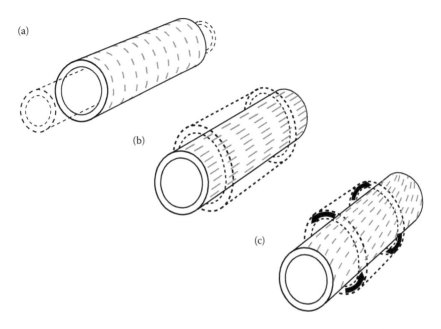

Figure 3.6 A schematic depicting a flexible water-filled elastomer tube with muscle-like actuators arranged in three ways: (a) The muscle is arranged circumferentially; when the muscle contracts the segment will reduce its diameter and at the same time lengthen to maintain a constant volume (hatched image). (b) When the muscle-like actuator is arranged longitudinally, contraction will shorten the tube and at the same time expand circumferentially (hatched image) to maintain a constant volume. (c) When muscle actuators that are arranged obliquely (helically) contract, they will produce a twist and contraction along the longitudinal axis (hatched image) at a constant volume. (Drawings by Iain A. Anderson.)

which were designed for standing them up on a sandy beach after unloading from a galley.

Starfish that live on a rocky surface have tube feet that are flat ended, which can chemically adhere to their substrate thus enabling them to hold fast in the strongest wave surges (Figure 3.8). A starfish can improve its hold on the rock by adapting its body shape to the irregular surface; the skeleton of the starfish is made of lots of little pieces of calcite (ossicles) held together by strands of collagen that can change stiffness. Thus, the starfish softens its collagen, changes its shape to conform to the surface, and stiffens the collagen again. By doing this, it essentially redesigns its skeleton adaptively. Starfish, which feed on bivalve mollusks, drape over the shell of prey, then by skeletal stiffening and holding on with tube feet can eventually open up the shells of their prey. The starfish then inserts its stomach between the shells and digests the hapless mollusk still in its shell.

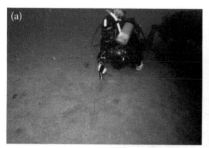
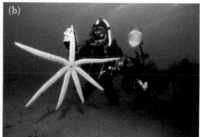
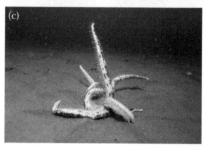

Figure 3.7 (a) Outline of a starfish that is buried in the sand, North of Auckland. (b) The starfish has been removed. These sand-dwelling stars excavate sand by moving their feet so as to fluidize the sand underneath them. (c) When laid down the starfish actively bends its body to bring the tube feet into contact with the sand. (Photos by Iain A. Anderson.)

Variable stiffness, conformable gripping used by the starfish can be applied to the design of tooling. Imagine a clamp with starfish-like soft and easily deformable surfaces that can be made to conform to the contours of a complex and fragile workpiece that can then be made stiff at the flick of a switch. Magnetorheological (MR) fluids can be used in the gripping mechanism. These fluids are suspensions of iron particles in oil. When subjected to a magnetic field the particles line up in the field and this increases the fluid viscosity that can "freeze" a mechanism. A design for a conformable clamp using MR fluids has been proposed. In this instance, the "ossicles" are spring-loaded pins in an assembly with an MR fluid. The pin array can be pushed against a surface and then frozen into position when the magnetic field is switched on; holding the workpiece firmly at multiple points [13].

For the starfish, each tube foot is hydraulically connected to a muscle-lined bag, the ampulla that receives water from an internal hydraulic system (Figure 3.9). A foot–ampulla unit is also relatively independent: there is enough fluid in the ampulla to extend the foot [14]. Like nemertean marine worms and numerous other living examples, the collagen fibers in the foot are arranged in a crossed-helical orientation [15] beneath which lies a "robust layer" of longitudinal muscle fibers [15]. Bending of a tube foot at a constant length requires coordinated

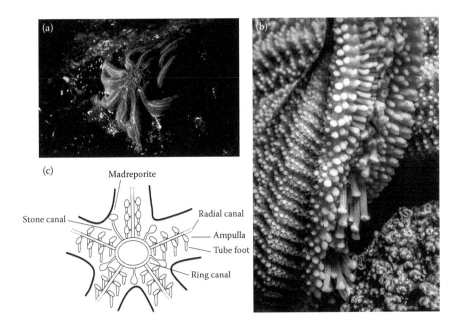

Figure 3.8 (a) A starfish clinging to rocks at Piha, Auckland. Water is filtered into the starfish's hydraulic system through the madreporite at the top of the central disk. (b) Individual tube feet can be seen in this image, some retracted and some fully extended to seek a footing. (c) Water travels along a calcareous tube called the stone canal to the ring canal that distributes it to the radial canals of the leg. (Photos by Iain A. Anderson. Drawing by Vivian L. Ward.)

muscle activity between the circumferential muscle that contracts the ampulla and the muscle of the tube foot [15]. Fiber angles must be greater than 54° (Figure 3.3) so that the foot will extend when the water is transferred from the ampulla; helical angles of about 67° have been measured on one species of starfish [15].

To the best of our knowledge, no one has produced a hydrostat tube foot on a robot that fully emulates the starfish. However, researchers at the University of California, Los Angeles (UCLA), have produced a walking multi-legged robot using artificial muscle "spring roll" legs. Each is capable of bending and changing length [16,17] (Figure 3.9). Spring rolls are composed of layers of thin dielectric elastomer membrane with flexible electrode on both sides, rolled over a precompressed helical spring. The spring provides support for the prestretched film as well as a passive antagonistic structure for the film to work against. The film itself is incompressible so that when electric charge is applied to its flexible electrodes the film will reduce in thickness and at the same time increase in area under the pressure (Maxwell pressure) associated with the electric charge. The film itself behaves as a volume-conserving hydrostat. Activation of the film will result in lengthening

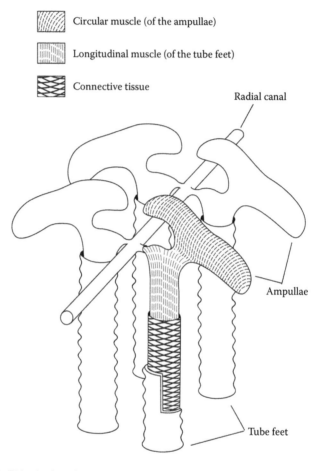

Figure 3.9 This depicts the local hydraulic muscular mechanism for the starfish tube foot. The lateral canals of the starfish hydraulics connect each tube foot/ ampulla to the system. Contraction of the circular muscle in an ampulla drives water into its tube foot. The crossed-helical arrangement of the connective tissue, at angles greater than 54° ensures that the leg will extend when water is pumped into the foot. Longitudinal muscle contraction in the tube foot can shorten the foot or bend it. (After McCurley, R.S. and Kier, W.M. *Biological Bulletin*, 188(2), 197–209, 1995 [15].) (Redrawn by Vivian L Ward.)

of the spring roll. Also, by electrically partitioning the film into two or four separately actuated sectors it can become a multi-degree-of-freedom actuator that can, in addition to lengthening, be made to bend about one or two axes. In the UCLA device one could perhaps replace the spring with a water-filled rubber cylinder with electro-active material wrapped around its outer surface. Such a system would then be a hydrostat tube foot: actuation would result in a shape change (Figure 3.10).

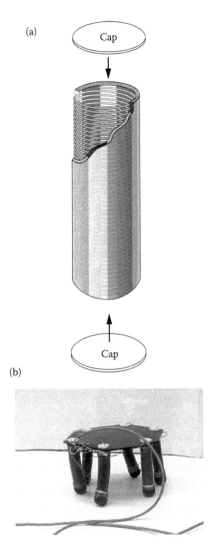

Figure 3.10 (a) Schematic of a spring roll design from Pei et al. depicting a spring roll actuator that consists of two end caps and a spring held in compression, covered by layers of an electroactive polymer (dielectric elastomer [DE]) thin film. The spring roll has four separate electroded sectors (darkened on the image). Activation of a sector will result in expansion of the film in that sector. This will result in bending. If all four sectors are activated the leg will extend. (b) A photo of a spring roll walking robot with 2 degree-of-freedom actuators. (Image reprinted with permission from Pei, Q. et al. *Smart Materials and Structures*, 2007. 13(5): N86 [17].) (Drawing by Vivian L. Ward.)

Muscle tissue is virtually incompressible as it is mostly water. Its living cells are full of proteins surrounded by an aqueous fluid (cytoplasm) that are joined to each other and to connective tissue within an aqueous medium. The perimysium, a sheath of connective tissue that surrounds the basic units of muscle, is also a crossed-helical system.

This opens the door to another opportunity: using assemblies of solid muscle to fulfill all of the roles of the hydrostat mechanism. If you are reading this page over lunch you are probably operating a muscle hydrostat of your own—the tongue. You can stretch it, roll it, bend it from side to side, and make it rigid, thus enabling the manipulation of food, production of speech, and expression of strong sentiments; poking the tongue out, for instance. But long before the tongue evolved, the cephalopods (octopus, squid, cuttlefish, and nautiloids) were using muscle hydrostats for their tentacles and bodies.

Muscle hydrostats are characterized by three "closely packed" muscle groups arranged in three general directions: (1) parallel to the long axis (longitudinal), (2) perpendicular to this axis (circumferential, radial, or transverse for instance), and (3) running in a helical or oblique direction along the outer circumference [18,19] (Figure 3.6). In the last instance, muscle fibers can take the place of restraining helical bindings that were described earlier.

Octopuses combine all three muscle types arranged in discrete layers and they can use their hydrostat arms to manipulate objects and build lairs for themselves lined with rocks and even capture fish! Several years ago, an octopus at the Monterey Bay aquarium was found to be hunting and ambushing small sharks. There are many other examples that demonstrate the octopus's problem-solving and dexterity such as reaching for a shell and the ability to unplug and open glass jars containing a tasty crab meal [20].

The key to muscular hydrostat operation is precise and sequenced actuation of muscle groups that produce lengthening, shortening, bending, stiffening (Figure 3.11), and torsion of the arm [18]. For example, contraction of muscle groups that are not aligned with the long axis of the hydrostat will result in elongation. In the octopus arm this could include the transverse muscles and the muscles running oblique to the long axis. Contraction of the longitudinal muscles combined with relaxation of the transverse and oblique muscles will shorten the arm. Contraction of longitudinal muscles to one side will produce effective bending only if accompanied by co-contraction of muscles that control diameter—the transverse and oblique muscles. If longitudinal and transverse muscle contract together the arm will stiffen. Perhaps the most tantalizing feature of the muscular hydrostat is the ability to produce torsion. This is not possible without active oblique fibers in the structure. Contraction of fibers arranged in a left-handed helix will produce clockwise torsion and vice versa [18].

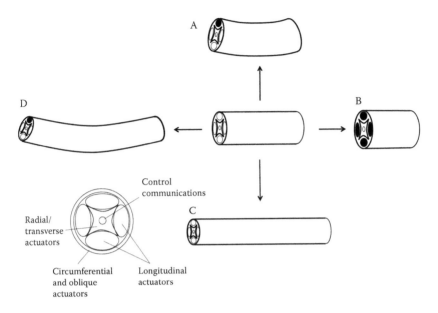

Figure 3.11 A concept muscle hydrostat mechanism based on the octopus arm. In this arm four separate bundles of longitudinal, muscle-like actuators are arranged at 90° to each other around a central control and communication cord (e.g., nerve cord). Also within the mechanism are muscle-like actuators that can contract in the radial and transverse directions. An active skin contains muscle-like actuators that contract circumferentially and obliquely. In A, one bundle of longitudinal actuators contract. Radial and transverse actuators also contract so that the overall length remains unchanged. In B, all four longitudinal muscle-like actuators contract, shortening the mechanism and causing it to expand radially to maintain a constant volume. In C, the outer circumferential muscle actuators contract and this results in lengthening. In D, the circumferential muscles are contracted along with one group of longitudinal muscles resulting in both lengthening and bending. (Drawings by Iain A. Anderson.)

With such a versatile and complex actuator there comes a cost in control hardware and processing of sensory data. There is effectively an infinite number of ways to sequence and activate muscle groups to enable a soft arm to complete a task such as reaching out and fetching an object. In engineering terms we can say that the octopus arm is hyper-redundant with respect to degrees of freedom. Compare this with our "human" arm that is supported by a rigid bony skeleton with joints at the shoulder, elbow, and wrist. The shoulder joint can move in three directions and rotate through three angles (yaw, pitch, roll). The elbow can move in one angle only, pitch, and the wrist can rotate in the three angles; only 10 degrees of freedom for our control system to deal with!

There are strategies for controlling hyper-redundant structures like the octopus arm. One lies in distributing control; a hyper-redundant robotic arm can have its own sophisticated sensors and local controllers that also transmit sensory and motor information signals to and from the central processor (e.g., brain). The other is in the use of a set of standard localized patterns of movement—the so-called stereotypical movements [21]—that also reduce the computational burden of movement on the central processor. The octopus uses stereotypical movements: a bend in the arm that propagates from the body to the tip will extend the arm in a closely controlled way [21] (Figure 3.12). Perhaps, the most remarkable strategy is to produce a pseudo-joint in the arm mimicking the operation of the vertebrate arm [22].

Several groups have been engaged in building octopus arm robots. Researchers at Clemson University and Penn State have explored the use of McKibben air muscles in octopus arm multi-segmented manipulators [23]. Hardware for an octopus-arm robot has been under development, led by researchers at Scuola Superiore Sant'Anna in Pisa (Italy) and the University of Reading (UK) [24,25]. The arm has a silicone body and utilizes embedded cables that are attached to servomotors to effect motion. The skin covering the arm has to stretch properly, else the arm cannot move so freely. The Reading team found that a composite material comprising a knitted nylon textile, embedded in silicone rubber, works very well and allows plenty of movement with superior mechanical performance [26].

The octopus arm can manipulate objects mainly because of the suckers. At sea level and with no water in the interface, the maximum force that a sucker can exert can be no more than the pressure of 1 atmosphere, that is, 0.1 MPa. An artificial sucker, inspired by the semi-passive suckers of squid was designed and manufactured by the Reading team. The sucker was about 7 mm in diameter, generating a lifting force of about 4 N at normal atmospheric pressure [27], or about 0.08 MPa, which is 80% efficient. Very impressive, and it is likely that the real thing, with its soft seal around the edges, can reach even higher efficiency.

Operating in water boosts the efficacy of an octopus sucker. Water is very cohesive, resistant to expansion as it is also resistant to compression. For the immersed octopus or squid, water lies between the sucker and the substrate and if you try to pull the sucker away the water in between will resist this. However, the bond will break when the pressure beneath the sucker reaches the cavitation pressure for water; this is when microscopic gas bubbles form within it. Pressures of magnitude greater than 2 atmospheres below ambient have been measured for an octopus [28]. The holding force also increases with ambient pressure so that for every 10 m we go beneath the surface of the sea, another atmosphere is added to this maximum force. Thus, cephalopod suckers become more effective with depth, providing formidable grappling tools for their owners. Perhaps this is why deep-water cephalopods have smaller suckers than their shallow water cousins.

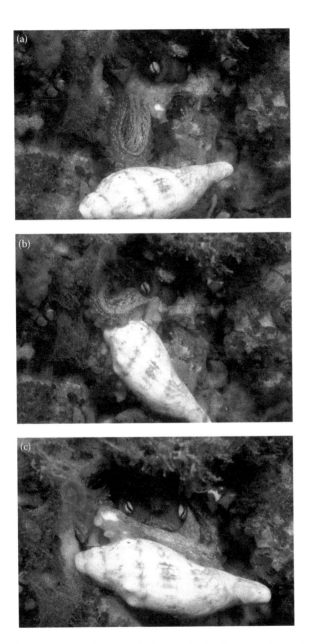

Figure 3.12 An octopus in a bay off of New Zealand's Coromandel Peninsula reaches out to grab a shell that it will use to hide behind. (a) A single tentacle is rolled out until it comes into contact with a shell. (b) With suckers attached to the shell, the arm is bent, producing virtual hinges so that the shell is drawn upward. (c) With further manipulation it becomes a shield. (Photos by Iain A. Anderson.)

On the engineering side, work is continuing not only to develop improved soft robotic device architectures based on cephalopod arms, but also to establish means for better actuation, sensing, and control [29]. Designers of soft octopus-like hydrostat arms should not lose sight of the need for feedback data to a controller. This would require sensing in separate sectors of the robot including the robotic suckers. Soft polymer sensors based on the dielectric elastomer could one day fill this role as sensors and actuators in a solid-state rubbery robot [10]. Or, they can be used as sensors directly on McKibben artificial muscle actuators [30].

With further advances in soft robotics we will soon realize the goal of a fully soft, controllable robotic hydrostat manipulator. Like its living examples, such a manipulator could extend several hundred percent, reach around corners and perform dexterous tasks for marine salvage, through to surgery.

References

1. Fine, R.A. and Millero, F.J. Compressibility of water as a function of temperature and pressure. *Journal of Chemical Physics*, 1973. 59(10): 5529–5536.
2. Koehl, M.A.R. Mechanical diversity of connective tissue of the body wall of sea anemones. *Journal of Experimental Biology*, 1977. 69: 107–135.
3. Shadwick, R.E. Foundations of animal hydraulics: Geodesic fibres control the shape of soft bodied animals. *Journal of Experimental Biology*, 2008. 211(3): 289–291.
4. Clark, R.B. and Cowey, J.B. Factors controlling the change of shape of certain nemertean and turbellarian worms. *Journal of Experimental Biology*, 1958. 35(4): 731–748.
5. Wainwright, S.A. *Axis and Circumference: The Cylindrical Shape of Plants and Animals.* 1988, Cambridge, MA: Harvard University Press. 132 pp.
6. Daerden, F. and Lefeber, D. Pneumatic artificial muscles: Actuators for robotics and automation. *European Journal of Mechanical and Environmental Engineering*, 2002. 47(1): 10–21.
7. Tiwari, R., Meller, M.A., Wajcs, K.B., Moses, C., Reveles, I., and Garcia, E. Hydraulic artificial muscles. *Journal of Intelligent Material Systems and Structures*, 2012. 23(3): 301–312.
8. Wainwright, S.A., Vosburgh, F., and Hebrank, J.H. Shark skin: Function in locomotion. *Science*, 1978. 202(4369): 747–749.
9. Pelrine, R., Kornbluh, R., Pei, Q., and Joseph, J. High-speed electrically actuated elastomers with strain greater than 100%. *Science*, 2000. 287(5454): 836–839.
10. Anderson, I.A., Gisby, T.A., McKay, T.G., O'Brien, B.M., and Calius, E.P. Multifunctional dielectric elastomer artificial muscles for soft and smart machines. *Journal of Applied Physics*, 2012. 112(4): 041101.
11. Potz, M., Artusi, M., Soleimani, M., Menon, C., Cocuzza, S., and Debei, S. Rolling dielectric elastomer actuator with bulged cylindrical shape. *Smart Materials and Structures*, 2010. 19(12): 127001.
12. Jordi, C., Michel, S., and Fink, E. Fish-like propulsion of an airship with planar membrane dielectric elastomer actuators. *Bioinspiration & Biomimetics*, 2010. 5(2): 026007.
13. Menassa, R.J., Sears, I.G., and Stevenson, R. Magnetorheological Reconfigurable Clamp for a Flexible Manufacturing System. U.S. Patent Office. 2005. U.S. Patent #4204481 B2.

14. Smith, J.E. The mechanics and innervation of the starfish tube foot-ampulla system. *Philosophical Transactions of the Royal Society of London. Series B: Biological Sciences*, 1946. 232(587): 279–310.

15. McCurley, R.S. and Kier, W.M. The functional morphology of starfish tube feet: The role of a crossed-fiber helical array in movement. *Biological Bulletin*, 1995. 188(2): 197–209.

16. Pei, Q., Pelrine, R., Stanford, S., Kornbluh, R., and Rosenthal, M. Electroelastomer rolls and their application for biomimetic walking robots. *Synthetic Metals*, 2003. 135–136: 129–131.

17. Pei, Q., Rosenthal, M., Stanford, S., Prahlad, H., and Pelrine, R. Multiple-degrees-of-freedom electroelastomer roll actuators. *Smart Materials and Structures*, 2004. 13(5): N86.

18. Kier, W.M. and Smith, K.K. Tongues, tentacles and trunks: The biomechanics of movement in muscular-hydrostats. *Zoological Journal of the Linnean Society*, 1985. 83: 307–324.

19. Kier, W.M. and Stella, M.P. The arrangement and function of octopus arm musculature and connective tissue. *Journal of Morphology*, 2007. 268(10): 831–843.

20. Fiorito, G., von Planta, C., and Scotto, S. Problem-solving ability of *Octopus vulgaris* Lamarck (Mollusca, Cephalopoda). *Behavioral and Neural Biology*, 1990. 53: 217–230.

21. Sumbre, G., Yoram, G., Fiorito, G., Flash, T., and Hochner, B. Control of octopus arm extension by a peripheral motor program. *Science*, 2001. 293(5536): 1845–1848.

22. Sumbre, G., Fiorito, G., Flash, T., and Hochner, B. Octopuses use a human-like strategy to control precise point-to-point arm movements. *Current Biology*, 2006. 16(8): 767–772.

23. Walker, I.D., Dawson, D.M., Flash, T., Grasso, F.W., Hanlon, R.T., Hochner, B., Kier, W.M., Pagano, C.P., Rahn, C.D., and Zhang, Q.M. Continuum robot arms inspired by cephalopods. *Unmanned Ground Vehicle Technology VII*, SPIE Proceedings, Vol. 5804, 2005.

24. Calisti, M., Giorelli, M., Levy, G., Mazzolai, B., Hochner, B., Laschi, C., and Dario, P. An octopus-bioinspired solution to movement and manipulation for soft robots. *Bioinspiration & Biomimetics*, 2011. 6(3): 036002.

25. Hou, J., Bonser, R.H.C., and Jeronimidis, G. Design of a biomimetic skin for an octopus-inspired robot—Part I: Characterising octopus skin. *Journal of Bionic Engineering*, 2011. 8(3): 288–296.

26. Hou, J., Bonser, R.H.C., and Jeronimidis, G. Developing skin analogues for a robotic octopus. *Journal of Bionic Engineering*, 2012. 9(3): 385–390.

27. Hou, J., Wright, E., Bonser, R.H.C., and Jeronimidis, G. Development of biomimetic squid-inspired suckers. *Journal of Bionic Engineering*, 2012. 9(4): 484–493.

28. Smith, A.M. Negative pressure generated by octopus suckers: A study of the tensile strength of water in nature. *Journal of Experimental Biology*, 1991. 157(1): 257–271.

29. Trivedi, D., Rahn, C.D., Kier, W.M., and Walker, I.D. Soft robotics: Biological inspiration, state of the art, and future research. *Applied Bionics and Biomechanics*, 2008. 5(3): 99–117.

30. Goulbourne, N.C., Son, S., and Fox, J.W. Self-sensing McKibben actuators using dielectric elastomer sensors. *SPIE Proceedings*, 2007. 6524: 652414.

Chapter 4 Jet propulsion
for soft bodies

The open ocean is a habitat for animals with no hard skeletal parts that propel themselves using muscle-lined tissue to push jets of water. This includes millimeter-scale hydrozoan jellyfish and newly hatched squid to meter-scale giants such as the Lion's mane jellyfish (*Cyanea* sp.) and the adult giant squid (*Architeuthis* sp.). All provide examples for how we might use jet propulsion effectively for underwater vehicles.

Squid jet propulsion

The squid can reach speeds of 5–10 m/s, when being pursued by a predator [1], putting it in front of any living aquatic creature for its size. The squid's hollow bullet-shaped and fin-bordered mantle is streamlined to minimize drag. The mantle is composed of muscle fibers and connective tissue and ejects water when its muscles contract. The water exits from a steerable funnel through an orifice whose profile can be altered under muscle control (Figure 4.1). The mantle cavity is refilled through two orifices where the head joins the mantle.

Refilling is driven by several mantle-opening mechanisms. The elastic energy stored in its tissue will cause it to spring open. This is assisted by active contraction of radial muscles throughout the mantle, for the squid's mantle wall is a hydrostat mechanism [2] (refer to Chapter 3), contraction in thickness results in expansion of wall area. Mantle opening is also driven by flow. As the squid moves fast through the water, pressure differentials between inside and outside drive it open, which helps to refill the mantle cavity [1].

While hovering and cruising squids also use fins (Figure 4.1). But as its speed increases the predominant swimming mechanism becomes the jet; dramatically demonstrated during high-speed swimming when the fins of the squid are folded against the body [3].

For an analysis of jet propulsion we can temporarily ignore the losses within a drive mechanism like the squid's and the fluid drag on the body as it moves through the water and just consider the ability of the jet to produce useful thrust. The effectiveness of this can be characterized by a measure of efficiency. For this,

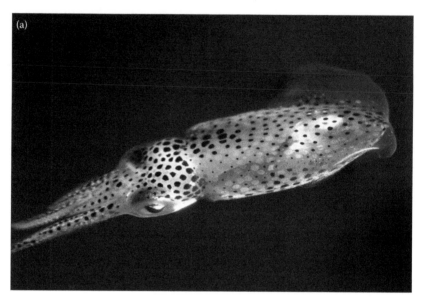

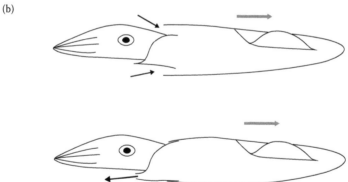

Figure 4.1 (a) Fins are visible in this image of a juvenile coastal squid (*Sepioteuthis australis*), hatched from an egg mass collected in the Hauraki Gulf, which is about a centimeter long. (Photo by Iain A. Anderson.) (b) Schematic of the squid propulsion mechanism. The funnel is closed as the mantle cavity is refilled (top). Water exits through a steerable funnel during jetting (bottom). (After Anderson, E.J. and Grosenbaugh, M.A. *Journal of Experimental Biology*, 208, 1125–1146, 2005 [3].) (Redrawn by Mark T. Ryan.)

the "Froude efficiency" [4] is often used. This is the ratio of useful power (the power driving the body forward) to the total power imparted to the water. This is not to be confused with the "Froude number," a ratio comparing forward speed to a wave speed. Both are named after William Froude (1810–1879), a British engineer and naval architect.

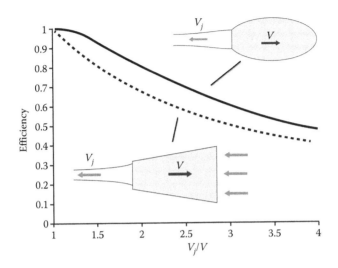

Figure 4.2 Froude and rocket efficiencies are compared. The Froude model (bottom drawing and hatched plot) is represented by a constant thrust jet-propelled submersible moving to the right at velocity V. A mechanism within accelerates the fluid entering the device at velocity V to velocity V_j. If we were to close the front opening and simply expel fluid out the orifice like a rocket (top drawing) we get something more closely resembling the squid during the jetting phase of swimming. The "rocket" efficiency is higher than the Froude efficiency. Both models assume a constant flow rate. This fails to account for the filling phase of the squid/jellyfish swim cycle and the changes associated with the pulsatile action. (Drawings by Iain A. Anderson.)

To develop an expression for Froude efficiency we can visualize a squid-like submersible that is continuously accelerating water in its path so that momentum transfer creates a thrust to drive it forward (Figure 4.2). The power that drives it forward (P_0) will be equal to the net thrust on the body (the difference between momentum flux at the outlet and inlet) multiplied by its velocity.

To obtain the Froude efficiency we divide P_0 by the total power.[*] This includes the power associated with thrust, P_0 plus the rate at which kinetic energy is added to

---

[*] Froude efficiency: The power delivered to the vehicle driving it forward is the flux difference multiplied by the forward velocity V: $P_0 = \dot{m}(V_J - V)V$. The rate of kinetic energy loss is $P_{KE} = (1/2)\dot{m}(V_J - V)^2$. The total power delivered from the propulsion system will be the sum of P_0 and the rate of kinetic energy loss P_{KE}. If we divide P_0 by the total power we get the Froude efficiency:

$$\eta_F = \frac{P_0}{P_0 + P_{KE}} = \frac{2V}{V + V_J}$$

the fluid P_{KE}. From this we obtain the expression for Froude efficiency (Equation 4.1) η_F, where V_J is jet velocity and V is forward submersible velocity:

$$\eta_F = \frac{P_0}{P_0 + P_{KE}} = \frac{2V}{V + V_J} \tag{4.1}$$

From this simple formula we see that efficiency will be close to unity if the jet velocity V_J equals the forward speed V. Therefore, a way to improve efficiency and develop useful thrust is to have a large volume of water jetted backward at a speed V_J that is not too different from the forward speed V. We can look to the design of jet airliners as an example application of Froude's principle for design. The older "classic" jet engines fitted to the first airliners such as the Comet or Boeing 707 passed all of the intake air through the engine, into the compressor, combustor, and turbine and then out through a narrow exit. More modern "bypass" engines pass only some of the intake air through the combustion chamber of the engine, but all of the air passes through the fan. The result is that this more efficient jet engine exhausts a much larger volume of air at a slower speed.

Water does not flow through the squid, rather it enters and exits from the same end, although there are separate orifices for this: one set for entry and a funnel for the exhaust. During the jetting phase of swimming, when water is forced out through the mantle, the squid more closely resembles a rocket (Figure 4.2).

A simple analysis results in a different expression for rocket efficiency* [5]:

$$\eta_R = \frac{P_0}{P_0 + P_{KE}} = \frac{2VV_J}{V^2 + V_J^2} \tag{4.2}$$

Equation 4.2 predicts the efficiency during steady jetting and it does not include the losses associated with filling of the mantle. This predicts higher efficiencies than the Froude model.

Constant flow is also assumed. This is clearly unrealistic, for squid (and jellyfish) do not produce a continuous jet of water. Instead they jet in pulses and they can control, among other things, the velocity and duration of the jet and the size of their exhaust aperture (Figure 4.1). To understand this better we need to study the dynamics of pulsed jetting.

---

* To derive the equation for rocket efficiency we take the useful power that drives the vehicle forward, the mass flux multiplied by the forward velocity V: $P_0 = \dot{m}(V_J)V$ and divide this by the total power: the useful power P_0 plus the rate of kinetic energy loss $P_{KE} = (1/2)\dot{m}(V_J - V)^2$:

$$\eta_R = \frac{P_0}{P_0 + P_{KE}} = \frac{2VV_J}{V^2 + V_J^2}$$

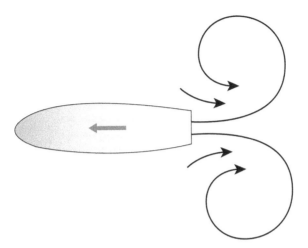

Figure 4.3 Surrounding water is entrained as the jet rolls into a vortex. (Drawing by Vivian L. Ward.)

The squid creates a turning mass of fluid, like a smoke ring (Figure 4.3). The phenomenon can be characterized by the length of the jet exiting the body L, divided by the diameter of the exit orifice D. Small values of L/D can result in nearly all of the expelled water wrapping itself into a single vortex ring. The jet will also entrain surrounding water into it [6]. The result is that a larger volume of water participates in the propulsion, and this is good for efficiency.

There is a physical limit to how much water can be wrapped into a jet pulse exhaust vortex. This has been demonstrated using laboratory robotic devices that emulate the squid jet. Typically, the critical jet length L is four times the diameter of the funnel D ($L/D = 4$) [7]. At greater L/D the vortex ring pinches off.

Squid jetting has been observed in a study of captive juvenile and adult Atlantic Brief squid (*Lolinguncula brevis*) [8]; small squids that are within the same family (Loliginidae) as the coastal squid in Figure 4.1 and that grow to be about 12 cm (mantle length). There are two modes of jetting: a short jet of low length to diameter ($L/D < 3$) that rolls up into a single vortex ring, and a jet of longer duration ($L/D > 3$) characterized by a leading vortex ring pinched off from a long trailing [8] jet. For a fast escape, prolonged jetting resulting in a high L/D ratio is preferred.

Robotic systems such as the "Robosquid" [9] have been used to study the dynamics of pulsed jet propulsion. The robot, that consisted of a piston, cylinder, nozzle, and a stepper motor in a streamlined housing, was used for studying the effect of duty cycle (the fraction of time during which water is ejected during a single cycle) and the ratio of the length of the fluid slug L to orifice diameter D, on swimming performance. High-duty cycle and low L/D are good, potentially boosting efficiency by 20%, when compared to an equivalent steady jet. This might be due to the thrust-boosting effects of an "over pressure" at the nozzle end helping to push it forward.

Squids offer clues on how to design and use pulsed jets on submersibles of all sizes and over a broad range of conditions: an individual squid develops from a hatchling swimming at very low Re to an adult swimming at high Re. An example is the giant squid (*Architeuthis* sp.) that swims at Re from 1 (juvenile) to 10^8 (adult) [10]. Newly hatched millimeter scale squid (Figure 4.1a) have fins, a mantle, and a nozzle, like their parents. But they inhabit a world where viscous forces are relatively large and where "burst and coast" swimming (jetting followed by prolonged gliding), as practiced by adults, is not an option. Young squid practice frequent jetting, bobbing up or down vertically and lunging toward prey. Their nozzle is relatively large compared with body size. Their fins are also smaller relative to mantle length than the adult. What is surprising is that they frequently produce jets with jet length typically 20 times the funnel diameter ($L/D = 20$). This would suggest that efficiency should be low. But if the flow is slow and broad (due to the wide nozzle) the efficiency can remain high. From measurements of fluid motions in the "jet wake" of squids from the juvenile to the adult, Froude efficiencies based on average movements of jetted fluid over a cycle have been estimated at better than 70% with newly hatched squid showing higher efficiencies than larger juveniles and adults; but when the contribution of the fins to propulsion was added, the overall propulsive efficiency for the larger squid improved [10].

Jellyfish jet propulsion

At the other end of the speed spectrum are jellyfish. They are slow but robust and provide design inspiration for low-power robots that carry instruments "capable of conducting autonomous surveillance over large distances for extensive periods of time" [11, p. 1]. Work to date has mainly focused on mimicking the jellyfish mechanism of swimming with its contracting muscle-lined bell. This has involved the use of shape memory alloys [11], ionic artificial muscles (ionic polymer metal composites) [12,13], and electromagnetic actuators [14]. In a groundbreaking demonstration of tissue-engineering [15], embryonic rat heart cells were plated onto a jellyfish patterned silicone backing material to produce a bilayer of cell and silicone "medusoid." Using electrical field stimulation applied by two electrodes to the fish tank resulted in jellyfish-like swimming of the medusoids. There are clearly a number of ways to mechanically emulate jellyfish but to understand how to do the job well we really need to look at how living jellyfish move water.

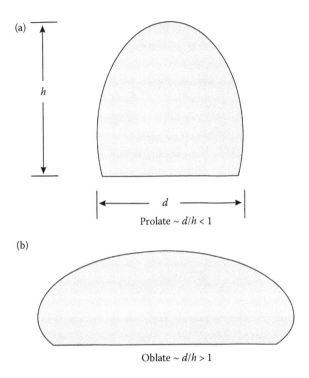

(a)

h

d

Prolate ~ $d/h < 1$

(b)

Oblate ~ $d/h > 1$

Figure 4.4 Jellyfish bells can be characterized by the fineness number: d/h, the ratio of bell diameter d to bell height h. (a) Prolate bells have $d/h < 1$ and (b) oblate bells $d/h > 1$. (Drawing by Vivian L. Ward.)

Jellyfish bells span orders of magnitude in size and come in a range of shapes. Perhaps the simplest parameter for characterizing bell shape is the fineness ratio (Figure 4.4): the ratio of bell diameter d to bell height h. The bell is prolate if the fineness ratio (d/h) is less than 1 and oblate if it is greater than 1. A species with a prolate bell is the hydrozoan *Turritopsis rubra* (Figure 4.5). They are small and you can sometimes encounter them in open water where they sit "fishing" with tentacles fully deployed, or in transit with their tentacles withdrawn and the bell actively pumping water. They are negatively buoyant so that while still and fishing, they are also slowly sinking. This brings them into contact with prey. Their profile, when contracted, could be described as a thick-walled cylinder, capped at one end [16].

Faster swimming prolate jellyfish (e.g., Cubozoans) contract their bodies over the entire length of the bell. And since the prolate jellyfish have a relatively larger cavity from which they can expel water they can produce substantially more thrust than the slower swimming oblate ones that contract more at the rim to produce a "broader, lower velocity jet" useful for circulating water and trapping

63

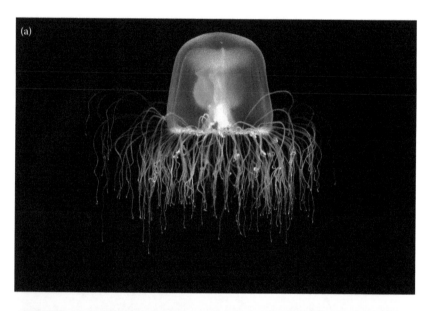

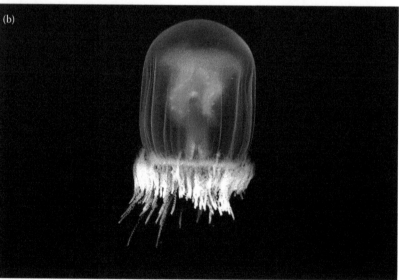

Figure 4.5 A hydrozoan jellyfish (*Turritopsis rubra*) from the Hauraki Gulf, Auckland. The tentacles are fully deployed in (a) and retracted in (b). After deploying its tentacles, the jellyfish will slowly sink while fishing for food along the way. (Photos by Iain A. Anderson.)

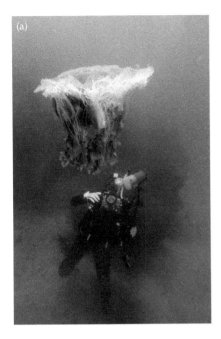
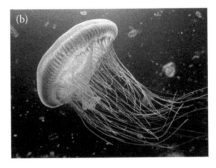

Figure 4.6 Two jellyfish with oblate bells. (a) The giant scyphozoan Lion's mane jellyfish photographed near Auckland. The bell diameter for this specimen was approximately 2/3 of a meter wide. (b) The hydromedusan *Acquoria* sp. photographed in the Poor Knights Islands is much smaller. Juvenile fish are often seen hiding between and under the tentacles of large oblate jellyfish like these. (Photos by Iain A. Anderson.)

prey [17]; a strategy practiced by the slow-moving giant scyphozoan Lion's mane jellyfish (Figure 4.6).

Coordinated contraction of muscles closes and empties the bell and so must be followed by opening and refilling, but there are no muscles that can do this directly. To open the bell, stored elastic energy is used, facilitated through elastic fibers, which reinforce the bell. William Megill in his analysis of a Pacific hydrozoan jellyfish showed how this can be done [16]. When contracted, the bell becomes quite thick. This stretches fibers that are aligned radially around the bell. The elastic energy from the stretched fibers can then be used to help the bell spring back open. The stiffness of the fibers increases with stretch during the end stage of the contractions so that it can more easily spring open when the muscles relax. The jellyfish can also take advantage of resonance associated with movement of water into and out of the bell. At the right frequency it will more easily overfill and the tension from the fibers that this produces can also assist in contracting the bell [16].

65

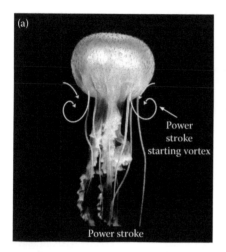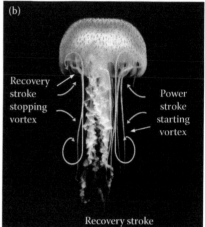

Figure 4.7 We depict two images of the scyphozoan medusa (*Pelagia noctiluca*). The vortices associated with starting and stopping are indicated in the drawings. (a) Water around the jellyfish is entrained during the power stroke. This will bring plankton food into close proximity to the tentacles. (b) Water enters the bell during the recovery stroke. *Pelagia noctiluca* and other scyphozoan jellyfish have flaps about the bell margin that assist with propulsion. They also have sensory, pacemaker devices (rhopalia) around the periphery of the bell. Rhopalia (white spots) are visible along the lower margin of the bell. The conduction system is hyper-redundant. The pacemaker signal from each of the rhopalia can travel by multiple paths to trigger all of the swim musculature. The first to fire initiates bell contraction and resets the other rhopalia pacemakers. (Adapted from Dabiri, J.O. et al. *Journal of Experimental Biology*, 208(7), 1257–1265, 2005 [19].) (Photos and drawing by Iain A. Anderson.)

If we are to seriously consider jet propulsion for an autonomous robot, one might ask: How can we make jet propulsion effective and efficient for locomotion? One way to improve efficiency would be to optimize timing of jellyfish-like swimming, divided between expelling water and refilling the bell. Rapid and short contractions to produce high thrust will require more energy and too rapid refilling can result in negative thrust: the jellyfish robot could suck itself backward. But if the period of refilling is too long then the average velocity will be low as the animal spends much of its time slowing down or resting. A modeling study has suggested that for maximum efficiency a phase-duration (time spent relaxing/ time spent contracting) of about 2 is ideal [18], although the model ignored other influences such as changes to the exhaust aperture during the cycle.

The Froude model (Equation 4.1) is also a poor fit for jellyfish: as for squid, jellyfish move in pulses. Also the bottom of the bell, serves both as water intake and jet outlet. Despite this poor fit between theory and reality a pseudo-Froude efficiency based on Equation 4.1 has been calculated for jellyfish, using averaged values during a cycle. In one study, four (hydromedusan) jellyfish were compared: two oblate and two prolate [17]. Froude efficiencies of the two oblate species were almost double the efficiencies of the two prolate ones. The oblate jellyfish has no rush to get anywhere and much of their effort goes into creating water currents past the jellyfish bringing prey into contact with tentacles.

A study of the vortex pattern created by oblate jellyfish [19] has revealed how vortices created during the power stroke and the expansion of the bell combine to enhance propulsion and feeding currents beneath the bell (Figure 4.7). While contracting during the power stroke a jet of water is expelled from under the bell and this creates a mushroom-shaped vortex that entrains water from outside the bell that travels downstream from it. This is called the "starting" vortex. When the bell relaxes another vortex is formed that rotates in the opposite sense to the starting vortex. This "stopping" vortex helps to refill the bell chamber. As the next cycle begins, the remainder of the stopping vortex that is ejected from the bell interacts with the starting vortex of the next cycle. This increases the volume in the next starting vortex and at the same time reduces its vorticity. The volume increase has a bigger effect than the reduction in vorticity so that the net result is an increase in the overall momentum transferred to the jellyfish.

Flexibility of the bell margin plays a significant role in the enhancement of swimming and feeding currents. Some jellyfish such as the one in Figure 4.7 (*Pelagia noctiluca*) have gaps around the margin. The advantages of a flapping bell margin have been investigated using robotic jellyfish [20]; it can substantially boost performance.

Clearly, we should not be too quick to dismiss jet propulsion as inefficient, particularly when it is pulsed or used as a broad slow jet that entrains the water around it. It has been used by ancestors of jellyfish, squids, and a host of other animals for over half a billion years. And there is the tantalizing option of combining jet propulsion with other modes of propulsion such as fin swimming, as this is what the squid does. That jet propulsion is in such widespread use in soft-bodied creatures suggests that we should seriously consider this for a new generation of autonomous soft-bodied robotic devices.

References

1. Vogel, S. Flow-assisted mantle cavity refilling in jetting squid. *Biological Bulletin*, 1987. 172(1): 61–68.
2. Gosline, J.M. and Shadwick, R.E. The role of elastic energy storage mechanisms in swimming: An analysis of mantle elasticity in escape jetting in the squid, *Loligo opalescens*. *Canadian Journal of Zoology*, 1983. 61(6): 1421–1431.

3. Anderson, E.J. and Grosenbaugh, M.A. Jet flow in steadily swimming adult squid. *Journal of Experimental Biology*, 2005. 208: 1125–1146.

4. Vogel, S. *Life in Moving Fluids: The Physical Biology of Flow.* 1994, Princeton, NJ: Princeton University Press.

5. Anderson, E.J. and DeMont, M.E. The mechanics of locomotion in the squid *Loligo pealei*: Locomotory function and unsteady hydrodynamics of the jet and intramantle pressure. *Journal of Experimental Biology*, 2000. 203(18): 2851–2863.

6. Ruiz, L.A., Whittlesey, R.W. and Dabiri, J.O. Vortex-enhanced propulsion. *Journal of Fluid Mechanics*, 2011. 668: 5–32.

7. Gharib, M., Rambod, E., and Shariff, K. A universal time scale for vortex ring formation. *Journal of Fluid Mechanics*, 1998. 360: 121–140.

8. Bartol, I.K., Krueger, P.S., Stewart, W.J., and Thompson, J.T. Hydrodynamics of pulsed jetting in juvenile and adult brief squid Lolliguncula brevis: Evidence of multiple jet "modes" and their implications for propulsive efficiency. *Journal of Experimental Biology*, 2009. 212(12): 1889–1903.

9. Moslemi, A.A. and Krueger, P.S. Propulsive efficiency of a biomorphic pulsed-jet underwater vehicle. *Bioinspiration & Biomimetics*, 2010. 5(3): 036003.

10. Bartol, I.K., Krueger, P.S., Thompson, J.T., and Stewart, W.J. Swimming dynamics and propulsive efficiency of squids throughout ontogeny. *Integrative and Comparative Biology*, 2008. 48(6): 720–733.

11. Villanueva, A., Smith, C., and Priya, S. A biomimetic robotic jellyfish (Robojelly) actuated by shape memory alloy composite actuators. *Bioinspiration & Biomimetics*, 2011. 6: 1.

12. Najem, J., Sarles, S.A., Akle, B., and Leo, D.J. Biomimetic jellyfish-inspired underwater vehicle actuated by ionic polymer metal composite actuators. *Smart Materials and Structures*, 2012. 21(9): 094026.

13. Yeom, S.-W. and I.-K. Oh, A biomimetic jellyfish robot based on ionic polymer metal composite actuators. *Smart Materials and Structures*, 2009. 18(8): 085002.

14. Ko, Y., Na, S., Lee, Y., Cha, K., Ko, S.Y., Park, J., and Park, S. A jellyfish-like swimming mini-robot actuated by an electromagnetic actuation system. *Smart Materials and Structures*, 2012. 21(5): 057001.

15. Nawroth, J.C., Lee, H., Feinberg, A.W., Ripplinger, C.M., McCain, M.L., Grosberg, A., Dabiri, J.O., and Parker, K.K., A tissue-engineered jellyfish with biomimetic propulsion. *Nature Biotechnology*, 2012. 30(8): 792–797.

16. Megill, W.M. The biomechanics of jellyfish swimming, PhD thesis, Department of Zoology, University of British Columbia, 1991.

17. Ford, M.D. and Costello, J.H. Kinematic comparison of bell contraction by four species of hydromedusae. *Scientia Marina*, 2000. 64(S1).

18. Daniel, T.L. Mechanics and energetics of medusan jet propulsion. *Canadian Journal of Zoology*, 1983. 61(6): 1406–1420.

19. Dabiri, J.O., Colin, S.P., Costello, J.H., and Gharib, M. Flow patterns generated by oblate medusan jellyfish: Field measurements and laboratory analyses. *Journal of Experimental Biology*, 2005. 208(7): 1257–1265.

20. Colin, S.P., Costello, J.H., Dabiri, J.O., Villanueva, A., Blottman, J.B., Gemmell, B.J., and Priya, S. Biomimetic and live medusae reveal the mechanistic advantages of a flexible bell margin. *PLoS One*, 2012. 7(11): e48909.

Chapter 5 Buoyancy

Most of us are near neutrally buoyant; it is relatively easy to keep one's head above water with a gentle kick. Our body is partly composed of bone, a structural material that is 2–3 times the density of water. The negative buoyancy of the bone is not quite offset by the 20%–40% of our body that is low-density fat [1]. It is partly through our air-filled cavities that include the lungs, trachea, and sinuses that we achieve near neutral buoyancy [2]. But it is the additional equipment we carry or wear that leads to problems. To stay warm we wear a buoyant wetsuit composed of neoprene foam, a compressed air tank that gets lighter as the air is used, and a belt filled with lead weights to counter the effects of the suit and tank. As depth increases the neoprene compresses. Close control of buoyancy is maintained through the use of a buoyancy compensation device (BCD); a collapsible safety vest that can receive air from the tank or mouth (Figure 5.1).

Control of buoyancy is difficult when both hands operate a camera. A sea surface nighttime encounter with a coastal squid by one of the authors (IAA) underlined this problem. The negatively buoyant squid ceased using its fins and muscle-powered jets of water to hold position and went into something like a skydiver's free fall with arms pointing upward (Figure 5.2); occasionally stopping to lunge forward at something in the plankton. Following the squid down, in total darkness, was initially quite easy but as depth increased the diver's buoyancy reduced.

With both hands on the camera, and concentration fixed on the subject, putting air into the BCD was not possible. All the diver could do to slow descent was to kick harder with his fins. The chase was abandoned, for safety's sake at a depth of 10 meters, leaving the squid to continue its descent alone. The BCD was then slowly filled with air from the tank to restore neutral buoyancy. As is standard procedure and to avoid decompression illness, a slow and controlled return to the surface was required, by purging air from the now expanding bag of the BCD. Purging it too slowly would result in a rapid ascent with the possibility of decompression illness.

The BCD mimics the fish swim bladder (Figure 1.10, Chapter 1), a flexible gas-filled sac that is located in the upper middle part of the fish's body that came into use with the first bony fishes approximately 400 million years ago [3]. Fish tune their bladders to give them neutral buoyancy at the top end of their vertical range so that a surface-swimming fish will be neutrally buoyant near the sea surface and a fish that lives on a deep reef will be neutrally buoyant at the topmost part

(a)   (b)

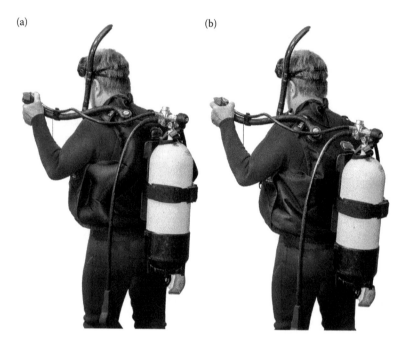

Figure 5.1 Photo of a diver wearing a BCD. The BCD is collapsible under pressure, like the fish's swim bladder (refer to Figure 1.10, Chapter 1). (a) The diver presses a valve that inflates the BCD. (b) The exhaust button has been depressed causing the bag to deflate. (Photos by Mark T. Ryan.)

of the reef that it visits. There is positive feedback between depth and density for soft-bodied creatures like fish and neoprene-clad BCD toting divers and this can lead to problems for both (Figure 5.3). It is possible for fish to adjust the gas in their bladder but this takes time. Few studies have been done on this problem, but the best figure available is that a reduction of pressure of 50% requires 12 h for equilibration. Therefore, fishes that live in deeper water cannot venture up to the surface too fast because if they do they risk bursting their bladder or becoming trapped at the surface. For a broad range for vertical migrations a small swim bladder (relative to the size of the fish) with a wall thickened to resist expansion of the gas is desirable [4]. Or one can live without it, like the squid.

Without a swim bladder, the negatively buoyant coastal squid (Figure 5.2) with its muscle-lined mantle and tentacles must swim to hold position. Swimming is not an important issue for active or shallow-water species like this. But for a creature that inhabits the open ocean, of average depth 2 km, neutral buoyancy could be an advantage. One solution is to use a rigid buoyancy device; a strategy employed by the deepwater squid-like mollusc *Spirula spirula*, which lives in just about all of the Earth's tropical and temperate oceans and seas (Figure 5.4). Evidence of their

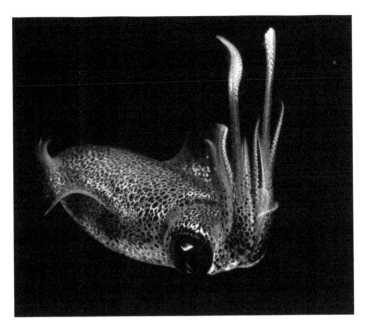

Figure 5.2 This coastal squid (*Sepioteuthis australis*), photographed at night off the Poor Knights Islands went into a free fall with its arms pointing upward. The squid, which is heavier than water can hydroplane like a submarine under jet thrust, or hover using its fins and a harrier-like downward-directed jet exhaust funnel or simply free fall downward. Coastal squid live over the continental shelf so they are unlikely to venture down more than 300 meters. (Photo by Iain A. Anderson.)

existence can usually be found washed up on the beach: a spiral shell, popularly referred to as the ram's horn shell, which is the internal buoyancy mechanism for the squid.

The life history and physiology of *Spirula* was studied in the 1960s and 1970s by a UK marine biologist, Dr. Eric Denton. In one of his scientific papers he describes how it manufactures the shell that is almost entirely contained within the body. As the mollusk grows it adds new chambers to the shell, forming the compact spiral. The creature's cells remove dissolved salts from the liquid within a newly formed chamber. The remaining dilute solution can now follow the salts down the concentration gradient (Denton called this "osmosis") leaving a void that is filled by nitrogen with a small amount of oxygen. The chamber is never sealed, however. The siphuncle, a cord of living tissue, extends along the spiral into all the chambers of the shell and so keeps the gas contents of the compartments under control, and allows water to reenter the chamber when necessary. The growing animal then begins the construction of a new larger chamber [5,6].

71

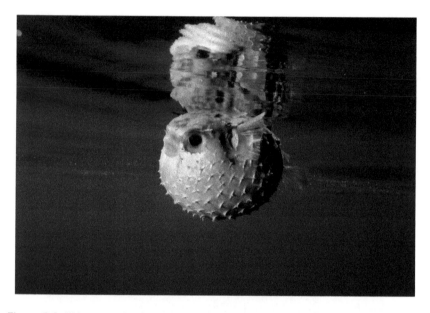

Figure 5.3 This porcupine fish (*Allomycterus jaculiferus*) with buoyancy problems was photographed floating helplessly at the surface off the Poor Knights Islands. Not sure why; perhaps it ventured above its range or simply swallowed some air. (Photo by Iain A. Anderson.)

The spiral design (Figure 5.5) offers a compact way of adding buoyancy compartments that scales with the animal. We could perhaps emulate such a structure: imagine a telescoping spiral buoyancy device!

The rigid gas-filled shell of *Spirula* enables a much broader vertical range than a swim bladder, since it can rigidly support a greater difference in pressure between the gas in the shell and the water. But if it ventures too deep the shell will implode from ambient water pressure. According to Denton [5], the shells of *Spirula* will implode at depths down to 1500 m although it is likely that they live above 500 m; a factor of safety of about 3. Still quite deep: 500 m is more than double the average depth of the continental shelf and well below the design depth for some attack submarines [7]. For submarines, the ratio between the collapse depth and the maximum design depth (i.e., the factor of safety) can be 1.5 or higher [7].

The *S. spirula* wall is made up of several layers of aragonite material (a crystalline form of calcium carbonate) that between them provide great stiffness and resistance to the propagation of cracks. The *S. spirula* shell has stood the test of time; and to make the shell any safer would require a thicker and heavier wall that would be less buoyant due to the shell material, whose density is over two and one half times the density of water.

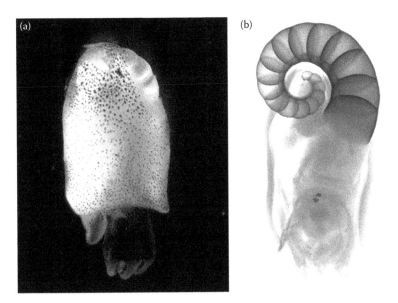

Figure 5.4 (a) The *S. spirula* squid is an inhabitant of the open ocean that relies on its rigid nitrogen-filled shell for buoyancy. (a) Photograph of a live specimen. This is how they sit in the water with their buoyant shell uppermost. (Photo by Dr. Steve O'Shea.) (b) A transmission x-ray image of another specimen. The two dark objects near the head are statoliths, mineralized masses that are part of the animal's statocyst balance system. (Photo courtesy of Auckland Bioengineering Institute.)

An ingenious variation on this theme was used for the Deepsea Challenger submersible that delivered the Filmmaker James Cameron on March 26, 2012, to the deepest part of the ocean: the Challenger Deep in the Mariana Trench; a depth of 10,911 m. The buoyant part of the submersible's structure consisted of a low-density solid/gas syntactic foam [8]: a ceramic, metal, or polymer infused with hollow microballoons. The foam, with a relative density of 0.7 gave the *Challenger* an upright "*Spirula*-like" vertical orientation with the observer pod at the bottom.

Neutral buoyancy can also be achieved by carrying low-density liquids. Some deepwater squid do this (Figure 5.6), as exemplified by *Architeuthis*, the giant squid that can exceed lengths of 13 m and tip the scales at over 275 kg. *Architeuthis* stores ammonium (a metabolic waste product), probably with chloride as the counter-ion, in its body, where it reduces the density of the water by comparison with the same concentration of sodium, the more common solute. Similarly, the smaller Cranchiid squids (Figure 5.6) have a special compartment in the body cavity, where they store ammonium. In both cases, the ammonium solution has a density about 1011 kg/m^3 [9], approximately 98.6% times the density of seawater

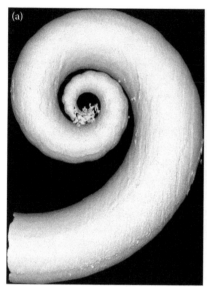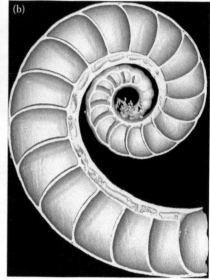

Figure 5.5 (a) A model of an *S. spirula* shell generated using microcomputed tomography. From top to bottom, as depicted, the shell measured 21 mm. (b) A cutaway view showing the chambers and the tube (on the inner edge of the spiral) that would have contained living cells that actively evacuated water from each newly formed chamber. (Courtesy of Auckland Bioengineering Institute.)

(1025 kg/m³). The Cranchiid squid with its stored liquid looks almost blimp-like, with the dissolved ammonium providing buoyancy to the squid, like helium in a blimp. It is also transparent. Perhaps this makes the squid hard to see as there are plenty of creatures in the sea that eat squid, but for us humans, ammoniacal squids are not very good to eat. The ammonia taste will curb the strongest appetite.

The blimp-like *Trieste* submersible, designed and developed in the early 1950s by the Swiss physicist and explorer Auguste Piccard, used gasoline for buoyancy. Although gasoline is more compressible than water (bulk modulus approximately half the bulk modulus of water) it has a low relative density of about 0.7 making it a useful fluid for this application. On January 23, 1960 the *Trieste*, piloted by August Piccard's son Jacques Piccard and U.S. Navy Lieutenant Don Walsh, made the first descent to the Challenger Deep of the Mariana Trench. The *Trieste* flotation hull (Figure 5.7) was over 15 m long and could hold 106 cubic meters of gasoline, which at a density of about 0.7 provided approximately 32 tonnes of buoyancy [10]. The flotation hull supported the much smaller but heavy two-occupant steel sphere; resembling a balloon carrying a small gondola beneath (Figure 5.7).

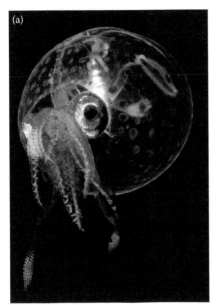
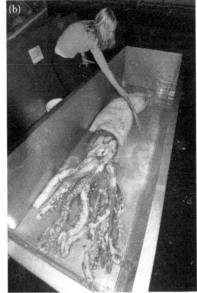

Figure 5.6 (a) Floating like a blimp, this New Zealand squid of the family Cranchiidae (*Teuthowenia pellucida*) stores ammonium, a fluid that is lighter than water and a waste product of its protein metabolism, in its body fluids. The 3 cm diameter squid was photographed at the surface off the Poor Knights Islands. (Photo by Tony Kelly.) (b) A female giant squid *Architeuthis* sp. caught off the Auckland Islands at 450 meter depth in a trawl. The mantle length was 1.8 meters with the mantle and arms together measuring 4 meters, and a total length with tentacles was about 12 meters. (Photo by Iain A. Anderson.)

Gasoline will compress more than the surrounding water and also contract as the temperature drops (the bottom temperature is close to 0°C), and given that the hull was not designed to withstand such high pressures, provision was made to allow water into the hull as the gasoline volume reduced; the immiscible low-density gasoline floated atop the water [10]. A much smaller steel sphere for the occupants of approximate mass 10 tonnes was suspended below the hull with a 9 cm thick wall and 15 cm thick acrylic viewing windows, designed as truncated cones, 10 cm diameter inside and 40 cm outside. Submergence commenced when two tanks at each end of the hull took in water, the ballast and craft could be made heavier by purging some of the gasoline. At the end of the dive, 10 tonnes of iron pellets could be jettisoned to allow the craft to return to the surface.

A key design feature of neutral density organisms is the near absence of stiff high-density materials, unlike the *Trieste* with its steel sphere and superstructure. The squids are almost entirely soft with hydrostatic skeletons. Another

(a)

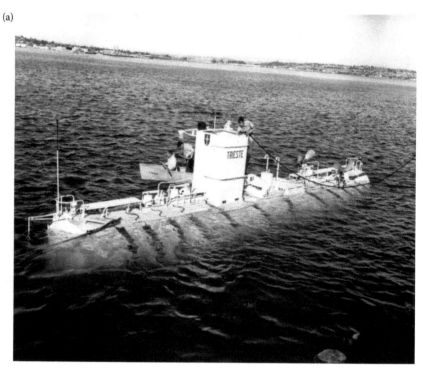

(b)

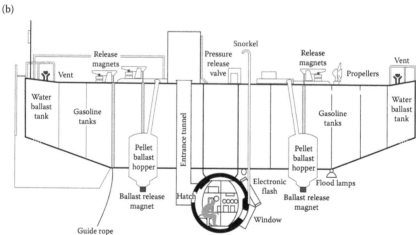

Figure 5.7 (a) The *Trieste* in the Mediterranean (circa 1957–1959), prior to the Mariana Trench dive. (From Vallejo Naval and Historical Museum via Darryl L. Baker.) (b) A drawing of the *Trieste* after the record dive to 35,800 feet in the Challenger Deep, off Guam, on January 23, 1960. (Adapted from USNHC #NH 96807 U.S. Naval Historical Center Photograph.) (Redrawn by Vivian L. Ward.)

example is the ocean sunfish (*Mola mola*) that has little or no mineralized bone in its skeleton. The sunfish habitat extends from the surface down several hundred meters and it can move up and down in the open sea because it has no air-filled spaces or swim bladder; using its prominent dorsal and anal fins for swimming and controlling pitch and roll of the body [11]. It has a very thick gelatinous layer beneath its skin and this, particularly for larger individuals, plays the major role in giving neutral buoyancy, being ~20 cm thick for one 959 kg specimen [12]. The specific gravity of the substance has been measured at about 1015 kg/m³ [12], 99% the density of seawater. A very large specimen recovered from the sea surface in northern New Zealand in 2006, probably the victim of a collision with a yacht, was a record 3.3 meters long and weighed over 2.2 tonnes with skin that exceeded 20 cm in thickness (Figure 5.8). Chunks of the skin that were cut from the body floated in seawater and sections of the skeleton were quite flexible and easy to bend.

Despite having a low mass cartilaginous skeleton like the sunfish and a large liver filled with low-density fats, the shark and its relatives, the skates and rays, are heavier than water. They also lack a swim bladder. If a shark stops swimming it will sink. But it can develop lift, like an aircraft using paired wing-like pectoral fins. And by swimming slightly nose-up, the shark develops lift with its body, like a kite [13]. Arching the body can assist control of pitch for up and down travel. The tail generates lift, too. Viewed from the side, the upper part of the shark's tailfin is longer than the lower part (Figure 3.5, Chapter 3). This pattern, termed heterocercal, sends water backward and down to develop both thrust and lift at the back end of the body, supplementing the lift generated by the pectoral fins and body

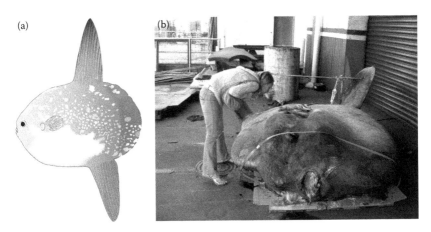

Figure 5.8 (a) A schematic of an ocean sunfish. (Drawing by Vivian L. Ward.) (b) This giant ocean sunfish (*M. mola*), found near Whangarei, New Zealand, perhaps the victim of a collision with a boat; it was 3.3 meters long, 3.2 meters high, and weighed over 2.2 tonnes, one of the largest ever recorded. (Photo by Dr. Steve O'Shea.)

[14]. And although the skeleton is flexible, the collagenous skin is an exotendon connecting the swimming muscles to the tail. Muscle support can be assisted by skin stiffening through the hydrostat mechanism that was described in Chapter 3. Thus, by moving the mechanical connections to the skin the shark can produce the forces it needs for swimming without the need for a dense and stiff structural material like bone. There is also the option of exploiting the advantages of negative buoyancy. Negative buoyancy offers the ability to soar downward underwater or perhaps perform a quick escape from a predator or underwater photographer.

In summary, a low-density gas, liquid, or solid can promote buoyancy, and gas is lighter than fat, which is lighter than water with controlled solutes. But all watercraft and water organisms travel to deliver goods, explore the depths, or simply to catch food. It is clear that the price paid for neutral buoyancy, whatever the flotation device, is increased volume. And with volume comes surface area and drag. The drag force for intermediate to large Reynolds (Re) numbers grows with the surface area of the body and the square of the velocity.

So, what price is paid for additional volume of buoyant material? We have estimated this using a simple model. In Figure 5.9, we depict an ellipsoidal submarine with length-to-diameter ratio of 4.5; a good aspect ratio for a streamlined body [15]. In this example, we imagine that the internal compartment is already crowded with equipment and stores and therefore the hull will need to be made larger by surrounding the internal volume with a hollow compartment that we fill with air or a low-density fluid to give the submarine neutral buoyancy.

The fractional change in volume associated with the new chamber V_{new}/V_{old} will be related to the density* of the submarine (ρ_{sub}), buoyant material (ρ_{bm}), and seawater (ρ_{sw}):

$$\frac{V_{new}}{V_{old}} = \frac{\rho_{sub} - \rho_{bm}}{\rho_{sw} - \rho_{bm}}$$

The amount of buoyant fluid depends on the initial average density of the submersible and the density of the fluid. The higher the average density of the sub, the greater the quantity of buoyant fluid. If, for example, the internal compartments of the sub had an initial average density about 2.4% greater than seawater

---

* V_{new}/V_{old} can be calculated as follows: When neutrally buoyant the mass of the sub (M_{sub}) plus the mass of the buoyant material (M_{bm}) will be equal to the total mass of seawater that is displaced (M_{sw}): $M_{sub} + M_{bm} = M_{sw}$. We can also write the original mass of the sub as the old volume of the sub V_{old} multiplied by its average original density ρ_{sub}: $M_{sub} = V_{old}\rho_{sub}$. The mass of the buoyant material can be calculated if we know its density ρ_{bm} and multiply it by the difference between the sub's new volume and its original volume: $M_{bm} = (V_{new} - V_{old})\rho_{bm}$. The mass of the displaced seawater (M_{sw}) is the new volume multiplied by seawater density ρ_{sw}: $M_{sw} = V_{new}\rho_{sw}$. If we put these three expressions into $M_{sub} + M_{bm} = M_{sw}$ and rearrange terms we get the equation for V_{new}/V_{old}.

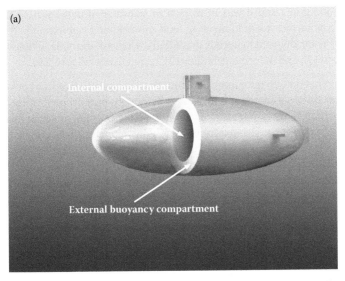

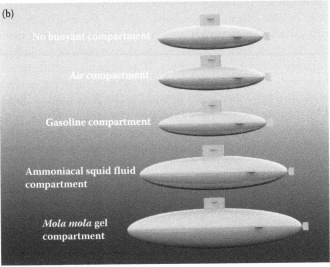

Figure 5.9 (a) A hypothetical submarine with an ellipsoidal hull. An external compartment is added that contains a buoyant fluid. (b) The submarine has an initial density of 1050 kg/m³, about 2.4% higher than seawater (taken here as 1025 kg/m³). The external compartment that restores it to neutral buoyancy must be very large for fluids similar to the squid's ammonium (1011 kg/m³) or the *M. mola*'s skin (1015 kg/m³). Here, we have calculated the size of the hull for it to accommodate the fluid. We have ignored the influence of the mass of additional hull material to carry the buoyant fluid. This would require even larger volumes of buoyant fluid to achieve neutral buoyancy.

(ρ_{sub} = 1050 kg/m³) and it was immersed in seawater of density 1025 kg/m³ the external compartment would increase total sub volume by at least 2%, 8%, 179%, and 250% if the buoyant materials that filled it were air, gasoline, Cranchiid squid ammonium [9], and *M. mola* gelatine [12], respectively (Figure 5.9).

Assuming that the sub maintains the same shape (same relative size between principal axes) the drag increase will be approximately proportional to the increase in surface area. This can be large depending on the buoyant material that fills the external compartment. Using a formula for ellipsoid area,* drag can be estimated to increase by 2%, 5%, 98%, and 173% to accommodate a hull compartment sized to carry air, gasoline, Cranchiid squid ammonium [9], and *M. mola* gelatine [12], respectively. To achieve neutral buoyancy for minimum drag a gas-filled buoyancy compartment clearly wins. But gases and some liquids such as gasoline are compressible. There will be a need for adjustment with depth unless they are stored in a rigid tank, like the shell of *Spirula*.

Being neutrally buoyant does not guarantee stability; resisting a tendency to "turn turtle" and roll belly up. For a structure immersed in a liquid, static stability largely depends on the resultant of the forces of gravity and buoyancy, their directions relative to each other (their vectors) and how the relative positions might change with attitude. An immersed body is also subject to pressure that increases with depth. Therefore, for a submersible, the deeper parts of the hull experience greater pressures than the shallower parts. If we were to compute the net force on the hull from each square centimeter of skin and sum these forces we would get a resultant vertical force that would be equal to the mass of the volume of water displaced by the hull: Archimedes' Principle. The position of this vertical force will depend on the shape of the hull and its orientation in the water. If the hull is composed of a homogeneous material then the resultant vertical hydrostatic vector will pass through its center of gravity.

In Figure 5.10, we have a schematic cross section through the hull of a submersible where we have placed an air-filled compartment to give the body neutral buoyancy. If we construct it so that the center of buoyancy (the point on the body where the resultant moment from the buoyancy forces [net moment] is zero) lies below the center of gravity any small angular deflection will result in a turning moment that will turn it further, a disadvantage for a submarine but an advantage for a fish.

The gas-filled swim bladder, located below the middle of the body renders the fish body unstable. A small deviation from upright position will also result in a moment to roll the body around further. But this static instability is useful for providing a gravity-assisted rolling moment and improving maneuverability for the fish.

---

* $S = 2\pi a^2(1 + (c/ae)\sin^{-1}(e))$ where a = minor axis, c = major axis, and $e^2 = 1 - (a^2/c^2)$.

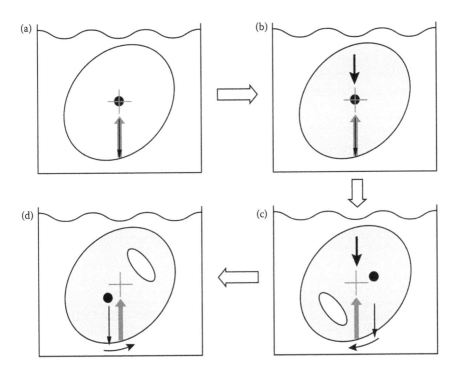

Figure 5.10 A thin submarine hull (wall material has equal density with water) with an elliptical cross section. (a) The hull is also filled with water, thus the water-filled hull's center of mass (black dot) and the center of buoyancy are coincidental. (b) If we now replace the water within the hull with a homogeneous solid that has a density greater than water, the center of gravity and center of buoyancy will remain at the same location but it will now be negatively buoyant. (c) We could bring the average density back to the density of the surrounding water by placing an air cavity within; placement of the cavity below the centroid of the cross section will result in the center of gravity being displaced upward and it will be unstable. (d) If the cavity is placed above the centroid then the center of gravity will be below the center of buoyancy. It will be stable. (Drawing by Iain A. Anderson.)

A diver carrying most of their ballast weight on their back and a full gas bottle that is heavy with compressed air can also be unstable in the same way. This is not immediately noticeable to most divers unless they take off their swim fins. One of the authors tried this (IAA), and was forced to hold onto seaweed, rocks, and pilings to avoid capsizing. The diver was like a top-heavy yacht without a keel. With fins on, the ability to resist turning was restored.

Thus a fish like the diver, must use its fins to maintain its normal attitude, which is why fish float belly-up when dead (this has not been tested on divers!). There are also dynamic instabilities that improve maneuvering ability for fish but these come into play when they are swimming forward. Each buoyancy mechanism whether by the storage of buoyant materials, or using a gas-filled float, or simply swimming forward has its plusses and minuses. And being just plain negatively buoyant like the coastal squid is not such a bad thing, for it makes escape easy from a predator or an annoying photographer.

References

1. Watson, P., Watson, I.D., and Batt, R.D. Total body water volumes for adult males and females estimated from simple anthropometric measurements. *American Journal of Clinical Nutrition*, 1980. 33(1): 27–39.
2. Donoghue, E.R. and Minnigerode, S.C. Human body buoyancy: A study of 98 men. *Journal of Forensic Sciences*, 1977. 22(3): 573–579.
3. Long, J.A. *The Rise of Fishes: 500 Million Years of Evolution/John A. Long.* 1995, Sydney: UNSW Press.
4. Jones, F.R.H. The swim bladder and the vertical movement of teleostean fishes: I. Physical factors. *Journal of Experimental Biology*, 1951. 28(4): 553–566.
5. Denton, E.J., Gilpin-Brown, J.B., and Howarth, J.V. On the buoyancy of *Spirula spirula*. *Journal of the Marine Biological Association of the United Kingdom*, 1967. 47(01): 181–191.
6. Denton, E.J. On buoyancy and the lives of modern and fossil cephalopods. *Proceedings of the Royal Society of London B*, 1974. 185(1080): 2730299.
7. Joubert, P. *Some Aspects of Submarine Design Part 1. Hydrodynamics.* 2004, Victoria, Australia: Australian Defense Science and Technology Organisation.
8. Murray, L. Cameron sinks to the challenge. *Engineering & Technology*, 2012. 7(8): 88–90.
9. Denton, E.J., Gilpin-Brown, J.B., and Shaw, T.I. A buoyancy mechanism found in Cranchiid squid. *Proceedings of the Royal Society of London. Series B. Biological Sciences*, 1969. 174(1036): 271–279.
10. Dietz, R.S. 1100-Meter dive in Bathyscaphe TRIESTE. *Limnology and Oceanography*, 1959. 4: 94–101.
11. Pope, E., Hays, G., Thys, T., Doyle, T., Sims, D., Queiroz, N., Hobson, V., Kubicek, L., and Houghton, J. The biology and ecology of the ocean sunfish *Mola mola*: A review of current knowledge and future research perspectives. *Reviews in Fish Biology and Fisheries*, 2010. 20(4): 471–487.
12. Watanabe, Y. and Sato, K. Functional dorsoventral symmetry in relation to lift-based swimming in the ocean sunfish *Mola mola*. *PLoS ONE*, 2008. 3(10): e3446.
13. Alexander, R.M. *Principles of Animal Locomotion.* 2006, Princeton, NJ: Princeton University Press.
14. Ferry, L. and Lauder, G. Heterocercal tail function in leopard sharks: A three-dimensional kinematic analysis of two models. *Journal of Experimental Biology*, 1996. 199(10): 2253–2268.
15. von Mises, R. *Theory of Flight* (first edition). 1945, New York, NY: McGraw-Hill. 629pp.

Chapter 6 Drag

Despite the use of thrust augmenting swim fins, a diver's top speed is only about 1 m/s [1], dangerously slow when compared with some tidal currents that can exceed 3 m/s and very slow compared with marine mammals such as the bottlenose dolphin that can swim at up to 6 m/s [2]. It is drag that slows the diver; but we can use it to our advantage: drift diving or traveling with a current can be an exhilarating underwater experience, as one passes rapidly over scenery and gets turned this way and that way in swirling eddies. If a current is faster than 1 m/s, the diver is virtually powerless against it. This can be frightening and dangerous if you are being carried away from boat or shore. One cannot eliminate drag but it should be possible to reduce it and be in control. To find a way to do this we can consider the factors that influence drag production.

Friction and form drag

Drag develops in a thin boundary layer that envelops the body, where water movement is influenced by viscosity: water's resistance to shearing or sliding over itself. The surface of the body entrains fluid, generating drag, and the greater the surface area the greater the total drag force from "skin friction." This source of drag combines and interacts with other mechanisms such as the drag associated with body geometry that is called "form" drag. The large resistance that you feel when you push a canoe or kayak paddle with its broad face oriented in the direction of travel is mostly attributable to form drag, arising from the difference in pressure between the paddle's front (high pressure) and back (low pressure) (Figure 6.1). Skin friction and form drag are sometimes lumped together in the term "parasitic" drag. If you turn the paddle 90°, the resistance will fall away dramatically as the paddle presents much less surface area and a more streamlined profile to the oncoming flow. Tilting the paddle further around at a small angle of inclination to the direction of travel redirects the flow of water and transforms the paddle to a lift-generating surface like an airplane wing. But with lift there comes lift-generated drag or induced drag.

There is a simple squared relationship between velocity and form/friction drag force. Every time you double your speed this force goes up by a factor of 4:

$$Drag\ force = \frac{1}{2}C_{Drag}\rho A V^2 \qquad (6.1)$$

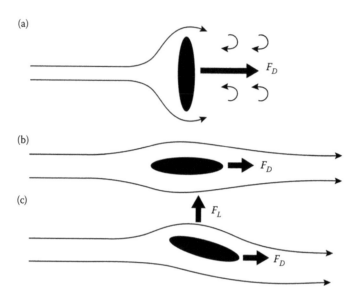

(a)

(b)

(c)

Figure 6.1 A schematic showing a cross section of a canoe paddle held still in a flow (or pushed at a constant speed) at different angles of inclination to the flow of the water. In (a), there is considerable form drag F_D behind the paddle; in (b), the drag is significantly reduced; and in (c), turning the paddle, which is at a small angle introduces a lifting force F_L. (Drawing by Iain A. Anderson.)

This equation includes a term for fluid density ρ and an experimentally determined coefficient: C_{Drag} that is referenced to an area A, which typically refers to the body's total surface area or its projected frontal area. For a wing or hydrofoil, A refers to the planform area, determined by the average chord length times the length of the wing. Using the equation for drag force (Equation 6.1) we calculate that to go from 0.5 to 6 m/s a scuba diver must develop 144 times more thrust force; a goal that could be well beyond human muscle capabilities! This is not surprising considering that the coefficient of drag for a diver ($C_D > 0.39$) [1] is more than 4 times that of some marine mammals [3]. The real challenge is for our muscles to generate the required power. Power is equal to force times velocity, that is, the rate of doing work:

$$Power = \frac{1}{2}C_{Drag}\rho A V^3 \qquad (6.2)$$

Equation 6.2 shows that if you double swimming velocity V, the power to maintain this goes up by a factor of 8! Too much extra exertion can result in breathlessness and the rapid depletion of air supply to meet increasing power requirements.

Parasitic drag can be minimized through streamlining. The goal for streamlined design is to reduce or eliminate the wake behind the diver, boat, or submersible. Two primary design considerations that relate to this are (1) the fineness ratio, the ratio of maximum cross-sectional thickness to overall body and (2) the location of the shoulder—the position along the body where the cross section is widest. This, as seen in most aquatic mammals and fish, is characterized by a head that is smoothly rounded at the front (reference the elliptical bow of a streamlined submarine), which becomes progressively wider at a shoulder region, and gradually reducing to a thin tail (Figure 6.2).

The wake is on average at a lower pressure than the flow at the front of the body and it is this pressure differential between the front and back that gives rise to the "form" drag. A cylinder has a fineness ratio of 1, and a very high form drag compared with streamlined shapes of equal thickness. In an analysis of airship bodies, Richard von Mises calculated the optimal fineness ratio [4]: "the stream-lined body of a given volume and least resistance should have a fineness ratio of about 4.5 and that even considerably more fineness, for example 6 or 7, will not appreciably increase the resistance per unit volume." For most aquatic mammals the fineness ratio lies in the range of 3–7 [5]. The fineness ratio (specifically the length-to-beam ratio) for the post-WWII fast U.S. submarine *Albacore* was 7.723,

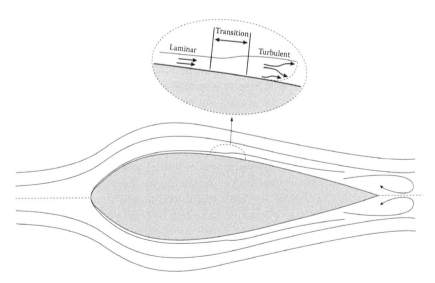

Figure 6.2 A schematic of a streamlined body in a fluid flow. The flow is laminar at the front tip and transitions to a thicker turbulent boundary layer somewhere behind the shoulder. The frictional tractions between body and fluid along with the geometry of the body contributes to the formation of a low-pressure wake; a downstream region of recirculating flow full of vortices that are shed by the body. (Drawing by Iain A. Anderson.)

and the drag coefficient (frontal area) was 0.1 compared with 0.35 on previous designs [6]. For fast swimmers, such as the orca, the fineness ratio is about 4.8 [7] and for the bottlenose dolphin approximately 5 [2].

Within the boundary layer, water can shear in an orderly way forming laminae, layers of equal velocity flow adjacent to the body surface, or it can be turbulent and chaotic. The flow can transition from laminar to turbulent somewhere along the body and beyond this point the boundary layer is thicker (Figure 6.2). The nature of the boundary layer, laminar or turbulent, influences the magnitude of the frictional traction between the water and the body—in other words, the drag. In a turbulent boundary layer, higher velocity fluid is pumped from the outer boundary layer toward the inner surface adjacent to the body's skin [8] (Figure 6.2). The average velocity gradient immediately above the body's surface will be greater if the boundary layer is turbulent, and because of this so will the frictional tractions associated with the fluid viscosity, producing a higher frictional drag force.

For a streamlined body, increasing its width up to the shoulder is favorable to maintain a laminar boundary condition at the front [9]. For swimming mammals at a relatively high Re, the shoulder is at least 1/3 of the way back along the body. The bottlenose dolphin has its shoulder 0.35–0.45 from the tip of its beak. The shoulder of a seal is at its midbody [5].

The transition from a laminar to a turbulent boundary layer is very likely to occur before Re reaches 500,000 (*Note:* the length parameter in this Re here is related to body length), somewhere behind the blunt nose of a streamlined body. Such values for Re are associated with flow along the body of many pelagic fish species[*]; thus the boundary layer along most of the surface of large fast-swimming marine creatures is turbulent. Data for gliding sea lions (coasting between swimming bouts) support this view. By timing their movement during coasting after a swimming burst, drag coefficient data can be obtained. Frontal area drag coefficient data for sea lions (where $C_D = 0.08$ [3]), are lower than the value mentioned above for the streamlined *Albacore* submarine ($C_D = 0.10$), but not by a large amount. At lower Re, viscous forces damp out any disturbances that might trigger transition from laminar to turbulent. At higher Re the likelihood of transition is greater. Surface roughness can also trigger the formation of a turbulent boundary layer [8]. And this can be beneficial since turbulent boundary layers are more stable than laminar ones; by this we mean "less likely to separate from the body."

Boundary layer separation results in a chaotic vortex filled wake and by delaying separation a smaller wake will result. Promoting a turbulent boundary layer might reduce wake size and form drag but skin-friction drag will be bigger. A frequently

---

[*] We calculate the Reynolds number (Re) (Equation 2.1) for a fish 0.5 m long, swimming at 2 body lengths/s (a typical fish swimming speed), and a water kinematic viscosity of about 0.000001 m²/s to be about 500,000.

used technique in wind tunnel testing is to place grit on the surface of a test airfoil near the leading edge in order to trip the laminar flow into turbulent flow and therefore delay separation [8]. There is "no pat answer" as to which is better, laminar or turbulent, as it will depend on the shape of the body [8]. It is clear that texture and form are inextricably linked when it comes to the subject of drag.

There is no doubt that dolphins are efficient and fast swimmers and there have been a number of suggested mechanisms for dolphin drag reduction. These include viscous damping of turbulence by dolphin skin, lubricious mucus-like secretions over the skin, reduced viscosity in the boundary layer through heating, and maintaining a lower skin friction laminar boundary layer by controlling the movement of water along its body [10].

Unlike the soft and flexible actively swimming bodies of fish and dolphin, watercraft are generally rigid and propeller-driven. Improvements in drag reduction have largely focused on design of the surface at the millimeter scale and smaller, using "roughened surfaces" (a catch-all for nonsmooth surfaces), to promote a turbulent boundary layer that will delay boundary layer separation. Early examples of such technologies emerged on the surface of golf balls, which were textured to reduce drag and generate lift from spin and the resulting Magnus effect as early as 1900. Analysis had to wait for the engineers and mathematicians [11], who tested a range of shapes of riblet in wind tunnels. Riblets are typically millimeter high parallel walls or more complicated shapes that are aligned with the direction of travel and capable of drag reduction of the order of 8%.

The discovery of the riblet effect raised awareness of their possible significance elsewhere. Sharks have riblets, in the form of denticles—literally small teeth—on their skin (Figure 6.3). The denticles are 50–500 μm across, depending on

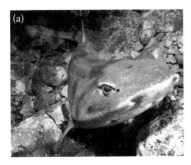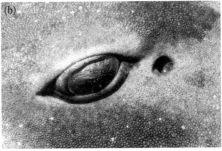

Figure 6.3 (a) A carpet shark (*Cephaloscyllium isabellum*) photographed in the Poor Knights Islands, New Zealand. This small harmless species, about a meter long, can often be seen resting on the bottom. Like all sharks, its skin surface is covered in denticles. (b) Denticles are clearly visible in the close-up view of a carpet shark's right eye and surrounding skin. (Photos by Iain A. Anderson.)

the species of shark. Amusingly enough, this caused a phenomenon that has frequently been seen in biomimetics. A physical or chemical phenomenon has been studied by physicists and chemists and (with luck) analyzed or modeled in the absence of any biological input. It is then noticed that a similar phenomenon occurs in a living organism and hailed as a biological novelty!

That shark denticles can act as drag reducing riblets has been demonstrated in an experimental study. A realistic denticle geometry from a spiny dogfish skin was cast using epoxy resin [12] and this was one of several surfaces that were compared in laminar and turbulent flows. The cast dogfish denticle surface performed better, demonstrating lower drag than a smooth and flat surface fabricated from the same material.

Riblets, in general, protruding from a surface increase the total wetted surface area and thus could be expected to increase drag. Two mechanisms have been proposed for how they reduce drag [13] (Figure 6.4):

1. The turbulent boundary layer contains vortices that operate in the direction of flow and crosswise to this. Due to crosswise motion some adjacent vortices combine their flow and this can lead to high-velocity bursts of fluid from the surface to the outer boundary layer resulting in greater drag. Riblets can impede cross-flows thus reducing these bursts of fluid from the surface of the body.
2. Riblets divide the vortices into two groups—those that are held away from the surface and interact with the riblet tips only, and vortices that are embedded between the riblets. Flow shear stress, which dissipates energy, is proportional to the gradient of velocity and develops between the first group of vortices and the surface of the riblet tips. But since the high-velocity vortices are interacting only with the tips of the riblets, the total shear stress is small. The second vortex group, embedded between the riblets (or denticles) may further reduce drag by rotating sympathetically to the boundary layer flow, acting like "fluid roller bearings" [14].

The questions then arise: Does the cross-section shape of the riblets and valleys have any importance? How deep do the valleys need to be (or, how high do the riblets need to be)?

This has been investigated in oil channels. Oil that was used, with a higher viscosity than water, allowed larger riblets to be tested for the same Re and better control of the geometry. Bechert et al. [15] conducted extensive tests on riblets with a number of different cross sections that included sawtooth (equiangular triangle) cross sections, and very thin rectangular cross-section walls separated by channels (Figure 6.4). They varied riblet shape, separation distance, riblet height, and evaluated drag for a range of Re. At very low Re the riblets reduced drag.

(a)

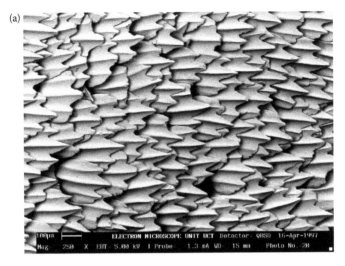

(b)

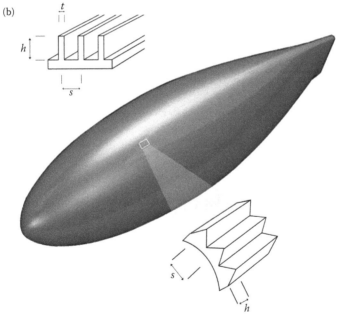

Figure 6.4 (a) A micrograph of great white shark (*Carcharodon carcharias*) denticles. (Photo by Dane Gerneke.) (b) Two riblet design concepts are depicted: thin rectangular cross section (top) and sawtooth (bottom). Here, we imagine cutting a small piece of a sawtooth riblet coating from the surface of a streamlined body. The designs can been compared experimentally by varying spacing (s), height (h), and thickness (t). (After Bechert, D.W. et al. *Journal of Fluid Mechanics*, 338: 59–87, 1997 [15].) (Redrawn by Mark T. Ryan.)

Drag reduction was optimal at a specific riblet separation distance (i.e., spacing) and fluid speed. Above this speed and/or spacing the drag reduction became less. At high speeds and/or spacing the riblets were detrimental to performance, increasing rather than reducing drag. Best results, associated with a drag reduction of 9.9% were obtained for thin rectangular cross-section walls (thickness only 2% of spacing) with height 0.5 of the spacing (refer to the "blade" type depicted in Figure 6.4).

Riblets have been tested commercially. In 1988, wind tunnel tests on a 1/11 scale Airbus *A320* largely covered with a riblet film showed significant drag reduction. In the following year, the film was applied over 70% of the surface of a full-size *A320* and produced 2% saving in fuel consumption [16]. However, when the film was used on aircraft in service, it had to be replaced every 2–3 years; the cost benefit was not realizable until the film had been in place for 5 years. It might have been possible to develop a more durable film, but this option was not followed up. Hence, the idea was abandoned and aircraft still have a smooth skin. Obviously if fuel costs rise, the idea will be reexamined. There is anecdotal evidence of the successful use of riblets in applications other than aircraft, particularly in sport where winning is usually more important than expense. The hulls of the U.S. challengers in the America's Cup 1987 and 2010 sailing competitions were fitted with riblets, were subsequently ruled inadmissible in the sport although it is impossible to determine how effective the riblets were. Riblets were also used on the rowing shells in the 1984 Olympics, but they were subsequently forbidden in official racing, together with all other devices that "modify the properties of the boundary layer" [17]. This is typical of the response of rule makers in sports—outlawing a technical breakthrough as soon as it is shown to be advantageous. The advantages of riblets on the sails of a yacht, increasing speed by as much as 5% [18]—seem not to have been noticed by the sport's stewards … yet.

Not all implementations of riblet technology are truly successful. Speedo, Inc. developed a swimsuit for competitive swimmers based on sharkskin designs, claiming that the Speedo Fastskin FSII suit reduces drag in water by as much as 4%. Oeffner and Lauder studied the swimsuit fabric under experimental conditions [19] and found no consistent decrease in drag. These results echoed those of swimming coaches who took a more objective approach to training their athletes. In the sports industries it is well known that you can improve an athlete's performance by hinting at the advantages of a novel technology. Athletes can be very superstitious, their lucky icons have the effect of making them more relaxed and confident.

There is, literally, another dimension to the sharkskin story. Shark denticles can hinge away from the skin, making them "bristle" [14]. This leads to increased vorticity within the water layer entrained by the denticles. These vortices might act as fluid roller bearings between the body of the shark and the flow. Bristling can be passive, due to reduced pressure above the skin, or due to tensioning of the skin during high-speed swimming [20]: stiffness of collagen increases as it is stretched, and the skin of the shark (which is highly collagenous) is stiffened by the sharks muscle hydrostat mechanism (refer to Chapter 3). Bristling might provide an active control mechanism for delaying separation of the flow over the body leading to a smaller wake and reduced form drag.

Wave drag

A boat or swimming animal at or near the surface generates drag when it produces surface waves. The general standing wave pattern that seems almost glued to the vessel, is the same whether made by a duck, near surface swimming shark, or a large ship. It is characterized by two wake lines forming a giant V with the vessel at the apex and with the wakes aligned approximately 19.5° to the direction of travel. Each wake line is composed of standing waves, one behind the other traveling forward at approximately 35° to the direction of travel of the vessel. The two feathery wakes are joined by a series of transverse waves of semicircular shape [21] (Figure 6.5).

The waves are gravity waves. In deep water (depth $\gg$ the waterline length L) they are dispersive; waves of different wavelengths (λ) travel at different "phase" speeds: $c = \sqrt{(g\lambda/2\pi)}$. Groups of these waves, originating at bow or stern constructively interfere along the 19.5° lines. As boat speed increases the separation distance between crests in the standing wave pattern also changes. This is very noticeable to the pilot, when the vessel sits in a trough of its own making. This becomes particularly noticeable when the ship speed results in wavelengths comparable to the waterline length L (Figure 6.6). For all surface movers—ships or dolphins—this is the "hull" speed, when drag due to the bow wave is very high.

The Froude number (Fr), a dimensionless ratio, can be used to establish the conditions when this will happen, typically the speed of the vessel divided by an expression related to the wavespeed. The Froude number is calculated from the vessel's speed, V, acceleration due to gravity, g, and length, L, of the body at the waterline or its total submerged length:

$$Fr = \frac{V}{\sqrt{gL}}$$

Wave drag can increase dramatically as the Froude number exceeds 0.4.

For submerged bodies, wave drag reduces as depth is increased and is almost zero when the depth equals the vessel's length. Wave drag can be a significant component of the total drag on a fully submerged streamlined body. Drag versus

(a)

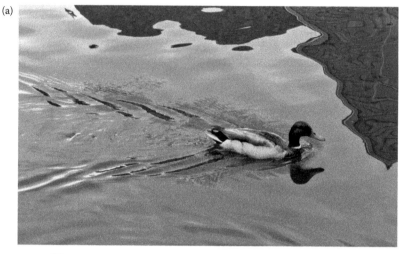

(b)

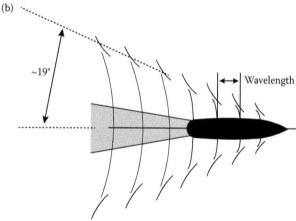

Figure 6.5 (a) The standing wave train that follows a surface vessel; specifically, a duck outside the Woods Hole Oceanographic Institute. (Photo by John C. Montgomery.) (b) A schematic of a wake pattern. The standing wave pattern follows the vessel as if it were glued to it. All surface craft whether it is a boat, duck, or submarine, traveling below the hull speed will exhibit this pattern. (A mathematical description can be found in Crawford, F.S. *American Journal of Physics*, 52(9), 782–785, 1984 [21]; Lighthill, M.J. *Waves in Fluids*, Cambridge University Press, Cambridge, UK, 1978 [22].) (Drawing by Mark T. Ryan.)

depth has been measured on euthanized specimens of the upside-down catfish (*Synodontis nigriventris*, Congo, Cameroon) that swims inverted (dorsal fin down) near the surface [23]. Inverted surface swimming is beneficial for this surface feeder. From near surface (immersed at a depth that is half a body length) to a depth equivalent to 2.5 body lengths, the total drag produced by the fish

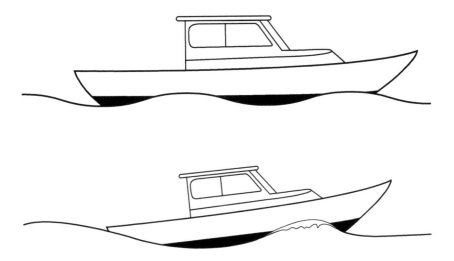

Figure 6.6 As the hull speed is approached, the bow wave grows in length and the boat sits in a trough between crests. (Drawing by Mark T. Ryan.)

bodies reduced to approximately half whether held upright or inverted (e.g., ventral surface up/dorsal surface down). Interestingly, the surface drag was about 15% lower when the fish were supported near the surface in the inverted position.

For aquatic mammals such as dolphin that must swim near the surface to breathe, wave drag is unavoidable. One strategy is to leap above the surface, traveling on a parabolic trajectory of one or more body lengths (Figure 6.7). This could be beneficial for efficient and fast swimming and would certainly reduce the influence of wave drag. Air has 0.1% the viscosity of water so leaping at fast speeds might

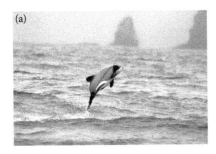
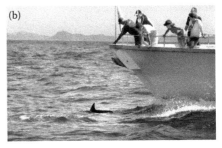

Figure 6.7 (a) A Hector's dolphin (*Cephalorhynchus hectori*) jumping clear of the water. (Photo by Michael Richlen.) (b) Bow wave swimming by dolphin (Northland, New Zealand). (Photo by Iain A. Anderson.)

reduce the energy cost of swimming. A study has shown that the crossover speed where leaping becomes energetically worthwhile is within the range of swimming speeds of dolphin [24].

Another approach to overcoming wave drag is to accelerate rapidly above the hull speed before a wave can build up. Although not a sea creature, the North American leopard frog (*Rana pipiens*) that swims at the water's surface is worth mentioning, for it has developed a strategy for fast swimming above its own "hull" speed. A frog swims by kicking its legs alternately or at the same time; the latter stroke produces twice the speed of the former. Alternate kicks produce speeds less than the hull speed but synchronous kicks allow it to swim faster than the hull speed, before the water can form a bow wave. This can be used by the frog for fast escape [25].

The boat's loss can be the dolphin's gain as it surfs the boat's bow wave or places itself where it can harvest energy from it by being pushed forward in the bow wave (Figure 6.7b). A small fish can also take advantage of the pressure wave in front of a larger fish: a manta ray or whale shark will often be accompanied by remoras and other small fish (Figure 6.8). Perhaps the bow wave can be used for underwater vehicle propulsion: this has been proposed for an unmanned vehicle that could be shepherded to its mission using the pressure in the mother ship's bow wave, riding it like a dolphin, remaining within the bow wave with guidance from a high-frequency sonar array [26].

Simply being alongside a larger vessel can be advantageous. Dolphin calves (less than a month old), handicapped by size and underdeveloped muscles, harvest propulsive energy by staying close to the mother's midside near her dorsal fin. This mode of swimming can boost speed by nearly a third and although it might slow down or hamper the mother's progress swimming alongside enables the infant dolphin to keep up [27].

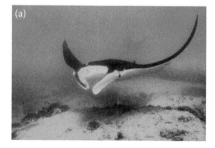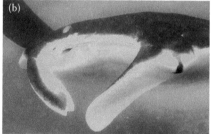

Figure 6.8 (a) A manta ray (*Manta birostris*) at Ningaloo Reef, Western Australia. (b) In this close-up, we see a flotilla of small fish maintaining position in front of its mouth. (Photos by Iain A. Anderson.)

Swimming near the surface provides an opportunity for harvesting wave energy. Packets of wave-driven water moving against the submerged flukes of large whales can provide propulsion that augments swimming [28], whether the whale is alive or dead! Whalers used this effect to help tow the carcass to the ship; and to stop it from drifting they cut the flukes off [28]. Wing-like foils that operate in a similar way can be placed at bow or stern of a ship and produce thrust from random swells. The idea is not new either; there is an 1895 patent describing this [29].

Thus, we have a number of strategies that can be employed to improve travel at the surface or beneath the waves. But where does this leave the poor diver? We cannot reengineer our muscles, so a good option is to reduce our drag. Students at Carnegie Mellon might have the answer to this, developing a vehicle inside which the diver's upper body lies; a streamlined and collapsible nosecone that includes a scuba bottle. The diver's feet protruding from the back drive the half-diver/half-submarine forward using a single fin with a dolphin kick. At the 12th International Submarine Races, a competition held biannually at the David Taylor Model Basin in Carderock, Maryland, they took the prize for a nonpropeller human-driven sub, recording a speed of 1.53 m/s (2.97 knots); substantial improvement on diver swimming speed! Perhaps such a vehicle could be significantly improved using riblets and improved streamlining. Then there's the prospect of strength-enhancing technologies: underwater exoskeletons that will boost our output and make us more at home in the sea.

References

1. Passmore, M.A. and Rickers, G. Drag levels and energy requirements on a SCUBA diver. *Sports Engineering*, 2002. 5(4): 173–182.
2. Fish, F.E. Power output and propulsive efficiency of swimming bottlenose dolphins (*Tursiops truncatus*). *Journal of Experimental Biology*, 1993. 185(1): 179–193.
3. Stelle, L.L., Blake, R.W., and Trites, A.W. Hydrodynamic drag in steller sea lions (*Eumetopias jubatus*). *Journal of Experimental Biology*, 2000. 203(12): 1915–1923.
4. von Mises, R. *Theory of Flight* (first edition). 1945, New York, NY: McGraw-Hill. 629pp.
5. Fish, F. Influence of hydrodynamic-design and propulsive mode on mammalian swimming energetics. *Australian Journal of Zoology*, 1994. 42(1): 79–101.
6. Joubert, P. *Some Aspects of Submarine Design Part 1. Hydrodynamics*. 2004, Victoria, Australia: Australian Defense Science and Technology Organisation.
7. Fish, F.E. Comparative kinematics and hydrodynamics of odontocete cetaceans: Morphological and ecological correlates with swimming performance. *Journal of Experimental Biology*, 1998. 201: 2867–2877.
8. Anderson, J.D. *Fundamentals of Aerodynamics*. 1991, New York, NY: McGraw-Hill.
9. Blake, R. *Fish Locomotion*. 1983, Cambridge: Cambridge University Press.
10. Fish, F.E. The myth and reality of Gray's paradox: Implication of dolphin drag reduction for technology. *Bioinspiration & Biomimetics*, 2006. 1: R17–R25.
11. Walsh, M.J. and Anders, J.B. Riblet/LEBU research at NASA Langley. *Applied Scientific Research*, 1989. 46: 255–262.

12. Jung, Y.C. and Bhushan, B. Biomimetic structures for fluid drag reduction in laminar and turbulent flows. *Journal of Physics: Condensed Matter*, 2010. 22: 035104.

13. Dean, B. and Bhushan, B. Shark-skin surfaces for fluid-drag reduction in turbulent flow: A review. *Philosophical Transactions of the Royal Society A: Mathematical, Physical and Engineering Sciences*, 2010. 368(1929): 4775–4806.

14. Lang, A.W., Motta, P., Hidalgo, P., and Westcott, M. Bristled shark skin: A microgeometry for boundary layer control? *Bioinspiration & Biomimetics*, 2008. 3(4): 046005.

15. Bechert, D.W., Bruse, M., Hage,W., Van der Hoeven, J.G.T., and Hoppe, G. Experiments on drag-reducing surfaces and their optimization with an adjustable geometry. *Journal of Fluid Mechanics*, 1997. 338: 59–87.

16. Choi, K.S. Recent developments in turbulence management. *5th European Drag Reduction Meeting*, 1990, London, England. 1991, Dordrecht, Netherlands; Boston, USA: Kluwer Academic Publishers.

17. Garcia-Mayoral, R. and Jumenez, J. Drag reduction by riblets. *Philosophical Transactions of the Royal Society A*, 2011. 369: 1412–1427.

18. Alving, A.E. and Freeberg, P. The effect of riblets on sails. *Experiments in Fluids*, 1995. 19: 397–404.

19. Oeffner, J. and Lauder, G.V. The hydrodynamic function of shark skin and two biomimetic applications. *The Journal of Experimental Biology*, 2012. 215(5): 785–795.

20. Wainwright, S.A., Vosburgh, F., and Hebrank, J.H. Shark skin: function in locomotion. *Science*, 1978. 202(4369): 747–749.

21. Crawford, F.S. Elementary derivation of the wake pattern of a boat. *American Journal of Physics*, 1984. 52(9): 782–785.

22. Lighthill, M.J. *Waves in Fluids*. 1978, Cambridge: Cambridge University Press.

23. Blake, R.W. and Chan, K.H.S. Swimming in the upside down catfish *Synodontis nigriventris*: It matters which way is up. *Journal of Experimental Biology*, 2007. 210(17): 2979–2989.

24. Au, D. and Weihs, D. At high speeds dolphins save energy by leaping. *Nature*, 1980. 284(5756): 548–550.

25. Johansson, L.C. and Lauder, G.V. Hydrodynamics of surface swimming in leopard frogs (*Rana pipiens*). *Journal of Experimental Biology*, 2004. 207(22): 3945–3958.

26. Ruffa, A.A. Bow Riding Unmanned Water-Borne Vehicle. U.S. Patent Office. 2009. U.S. Patent #8275493 B2.

27. Noren, S.R., Biedenbach, G., Redfern, J.V., and Edwards, E.F. Hitching a ride: The formation locomotion strategy of dolphin calves. *Functional Ecology*, 2008. 22(2): 278–283.

28. Bose, N. and Lien, J. Energy absorption from ocean waves: A free ride for cetaceans. *Proceedings of the Royal Society of London. Series B, Biological Sciences*, 1990. 240(1299): 591–605.

29. Rozhdestvensky, K.V. and Ryzhov, V.A. Aerohydrodynamics of flapping-wing propulsors. *Progress in Aerospace Sciences*, 2003. 39(8): 585–633.

Chapter 7 Fins and brains

Propelled by a giant caudal (tail) fin, the whale shark (Figure 7.1) that can grow 12 meters in length, comes up from depth to feed on plankton, cruising slowly, open mouthed, just beneath the surface. Although it can be much bigger than a noisy, propeller-driven, dive boat the shark is silent, creating no obvious wake in its path. When you see such a majestic creature you cannot help but wonder whether or not finned propulsion is superior to screw propulsion, used for all boats and submarines.

There are some clear advantages to finned propulsion: Fins can be extended or folded up and out of the way when not required; not so easy to do this with a propeller. Fins are also multifunctional. As well as providing propulsion they can be used for steering, and braking. Since they are manipulated in multiple degrees of freedom there are substantial control requirements for their efficient operation. This we will return to.

There are sound reasons for our almost universal use of screw propulsion. Propeller operation is simple, all that must be controlled is rotational speed and direction of rotation. Propellers are ideal for coupling to rotary motors and engines, and after almost 200 years of development, screw propulsion is reliable and also fast. On the surface of the sea, propeller-driven boats can outrun almost any finned creature. But when fully submerged the gulf between propeller-driven craft and the fastest aquatic animals is much less. The giant Bluefin tuna has been clocked at speeds of 15 m/s [1]; dolphins have been recorded at maximum speeds of over 6 m/s, some as high as 11 m/s [2,3], all quite respectable speeds compared with man-made vehicles such as the *USS Albacore* submarine, that pioneered the post-World War II adoption of streamlined and fast hulls, and that had a top speed of 33 knots (~17 m/s) when fully submerged [4]. If speed were to be measured as body lengths per second, the dolphin and tuna would outperform the submarine by many times.

Unlike rigid human-built watercraft, most fish and aquatic mammals are flexible, using their bodies and fins to swim (Figure 7.2). To swim efficiently there should also be as little kinetic energy transferred to the wake as possible. This is the basis for the Froude efficiency [6], η_F, which was described in Chapter 4 for a steady jet. Froude efficiency can be characterized as the useful power P_0, the forward thrust multiplied by the velocity, divided by the total power. Total power is the

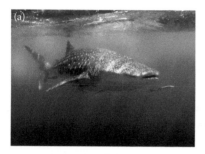
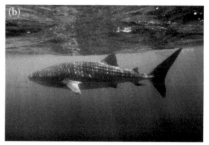

Figure 7.1 (a) A whale shark (*Rhiniodon typus*) at Ningaloo Reef, Western Australia, at least 6 meters long and accompanied by shark suckers or remora. (b) The body resembles a giant airship complete with a fabric skin supported by a rigid frame. This long-distance swimmer is distributed across the tropical and subtropical oceans of the world. Whale come up from the depths to feed on plankton, such as tropical krill. (From Colman, J.G. *Journal of Fish Biology*, 51(6), 1219–1234, 1997 [5].) (Photos by Iain A. Anderson.)

sum of the useful power P_0 and the remainder that is expended as kinetic energy imparted to the water P_{KE}:

$$\eta_F = \frac{P_0}{P_0 + P_{KE}} \tag{7.1}$$

To minimize kinetic energy transfer for the same energy input, it is better to push a large volume of water backward at a slow speed than to push a small volume

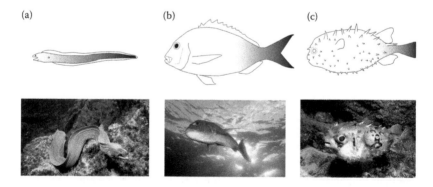

Figure 7.2 Three fish swimming modes are illustrated. (a) The moray eel swims in the anguilliform mode in which the body largely participates in swimming through its wave-like motion. (b) The New Zealand snapper (*Pagrus auratus*) swims in the carangiform way with much of the motion limited to the rear third of the body. (c) The porcupine fish (*Allomycterus jaculiferus*) is an ostraciiform swimmer. Forward thrust is largely produced by movement of its tailfin with little body flexing. (Drawings by Vivian L. Ward. Photos by Iain A. Anderson.)

of water backward at a fast speed. The small propellers of pleasure boats do the latter, although for a small boat it could be argued that this lost energy is worth the sacrifice if you can develop enough speed to get the boat "on the plane," thus substantially reducing its wetted surface and drag on the hull. With good design, high propeller efficiencies of the order of 70% [7] are achievable, given that some of the energy losses can be minimized using rotation inhibiting vanes or a counter-rotating propeller [7].

For fins to maintain high Froude efficiency it makes sense that they should be large and slow, maximizing the water that they come into contact with so as to provide adequate forward thrust without imparting energy to a turbulent wake. Unlike screw propulsion, fin swimming is oscillatory: the tail beating amplitude for fish is typically 0.1–0.2 times the body length [8–10]. Consider the tail on the whale shark with a top to bottom length, which is about a third of its total body length (Figure 7.1); with each beat the tail fin comes into contact with a large volume of water.

Fins are flexible and attached to a flexible body that, to a greater or lesser extent, participates in swimming (Figure 7.2) [11]. An extreme example is the moray eel, which uses a wave-like (anguilliform) body movement, ideal for navigating around and through very narrow rocky crevices. Open water swimmers such as the Australian/New Zealand snapper (*Pagrus auratus*) that swim in the carangiform way, using the rear third of their body to assist in the flexing of the caudal tail (as does the whale shark), are less maneuverable than the eel but capable of executing sharp turns, bursts of speed, and stopping suddenly. The much slower porcupine fish (*Allomycterus jaculiferus*), swims in the ostraciiform pattern with little contribution by the body at all. It is nevertheless capable of good maneuverability, using its fins to rotate its body and beat a hasty retreat from the diver.

Carangiform swimmers like the snapper are fast and maneuverable. At each beat of the tail a vortex is created that rotates such that its nearer part moves in the same direction as the tail. When the fish performs a reverse stroke, the next vortex turns in the opposite sense to the previous one and as the fish moves forward, a trail of vortices is left in the wake (Figure 7.3) that have an opposite rotational sense to those in the Karman vortex street; which can form behind a body immersed in a steady flow. In the classic Karman vortex street, the characteristics of the vortices at a given Reynolds number will be a function of the vortex shedding frequency f, the velocity of the flow V, and the cylinder diameter l. These three parameters can be combined into the nondimensional Strouhal number, St (Equation 7.2), named after Vincenc Strouhal a nineteenth century Czech experimental physicist:

$$St = \frac{fl}{V} \tag{7.2}$$

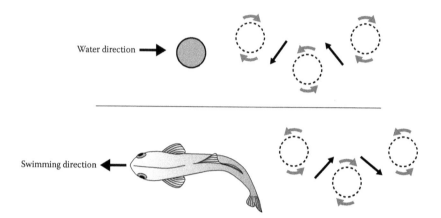

Figure 7.3 A reverse Karman vortex street produced by a fish (bottom). The vortices spin in the reverse direction to the vortices that form behind an object such as a cylinder (top) that stands stationary in a fluid flow. (Drawing by Vivian L. Ward.)

The vortex pattern produced by the fish, the so-called "reverse Karman street" (Figure 7.3) can also be characterized using a Strouhal number [12], where f is now the frequency of tail flapping, l the width of the wake, taken as the double amplitude of tail flapping, and V the swimming speed. For example, if a fish flaps its tail once every second and swings it side to side through a distance of 5 cm and swims forward at a speed of 15 cm/s it will have a Strouhal number of about 0.33. Fin swimmers from goldfish to sharks and dolphin swing their tails at Strouhal numbers in the range 0.25–0.35; by doing this they produce effective rearward-directed jets of water [13].

Dolphins and other fast open ocean swimmers, including tuna, use their relatively stiff tail fins to produce swimming thrust through the generation of hydrodynamic lift. This involves the side-to-side movement by the tail of a relatively stiff crescent-shaped (lunate) hydrofoil in a mode of swimming called "thunniform" (Figure 7.4).

A number of geometric factors influence the efficacy of the fin operating as a lift-generating surface. For instance, a high aspect ratio (AR) fin, where AR is defined as the square of the fin span b, divided by the total planform area of the fin A ($AR = b^2/A$) (Figure 7.4), is good for efficient swimming. For thunniform swimmers AR ranges from about 4.5 to 7.2 [11]. Another geometric innovation includes the use of tubercles [14]; leading edge bumps as seen on the giant flippers of the humpback whale (*Megaptera novaeangliae*), the only baleen whale that relies on maneuverability to capture prey (Figure 7.5). The long flippers of the humpback

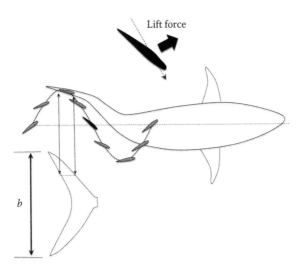

Figure 7.4 A thunniform swimmer is depicted. The horizontal position of a section through its relatively stiff lunate tail is shown through one swimming cycle. The black cross section is magnified to illustrate the forward-pointing direction for the lift force that contributes to forward thrust. A side view of the lunate tail is displayed at the bottom. (After Sfakiotakis, M., Lane, D.M., and Davies, J.B.C. *IEEE Journal of Oceanic Engineering*, 24(2), 1999 [11].) (Drawing by Iain A. Anderson.)

develop lift that enables the whale to do tight turns and other aquabatic maneuvers while corralling their plankton prey within a "bubble" net, blown by the whale. To maintain tight turns they must avoid a stall; a phenomenon associated with abrupt boundary layer separation from the wing when a critical angle of attack to the fluid flow is exceeded. The tubercles that line the leading edge of the fins have a demonstrated capacity to delay a stall while at the same time, increasing lift and reducing drag [15].

Returning to the lunate tail, a tail cross section has an airfoil shape so we could be tempted to try to estimate how much forward thrust the tail section produces using airfoil theory: by finding an equivalent NACA* airfoil shape. Using published lift and drag coefficients for an appropriate Re and the correct angle of attack of airfoil (the angle between the chord line and the oncoming flow) we can then calculate the thrust that this will produce.

---

* NACA refers to the National Advisory Committee for Aeronautics, a U.S. federal agency that was founded in 1915 to foster and provide aeronautical science. In 1958, this organization became the U.S. National Aeronautics and Space Administration.

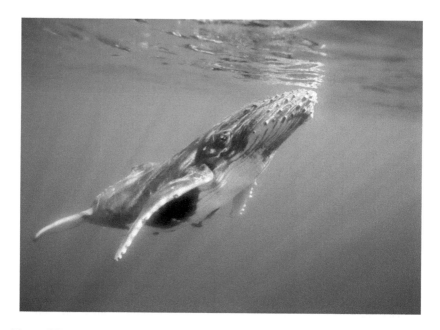

Figure 7.5 The tubercles are clearly visible on this humpback whale (*Megaptera novaeangliae*) photographed in Tonga. (From Fish, F.E. et al. *Integrative and Comparative Biology*, 51(1), 203–213, 2011 [14].) (Photo by Kim Westerskov.)

But NACA data relate to closely controlled drag and lift force measurements on a wing section in a wind tunnel where the flow is steady. For the fish, the situation is more complicated due to the unsteady nature of tail motion. In each cycle the flow across the fin is continually changing. This includes changes in the angle of attack; most extreme when the fin reaches one end of its travel and reverses direction. As the fin starts its return to the centerline, the flow settles and the lift-developing capacity improves until the fin reaches the opposite side and reverses direction again [16].

Oscillatory fish-like swimming has been studied using a range of mechanisms from closely controlled single fin devices to complex robotic fish. Perhaps the simplest way to produce thrust involves rotating a streamlined body around a single axis along its chord line. Sailors in one-person sailing dinghies might do this with their rudders when there is no wind by pulling the tiller to left and right so that the rudder is made to flap in a sculling motion. Researchers at Bath University have shown that it is beneficial for such a reciprocating fin propulsor to be flexible and that the distribution of stiffness along the fin is an important determinant of its ability to generate thrust. They measured the forces produced by flexible rubber fins that were rotated along an axis 10% of the cord-line from the front. Their biomimetic fin that had a similar stiffness distribution to the body of a pumpkinseed sunfish (*Lepomis gibbosus*) was compared with a fin based on the NACA0012* airfoil profile. The rubber biomimetic design was thicker than the NACA0012 profile at the quarter chord (25% behind the tip) and tapered to a much thinner cross section behind this. Their biomimetic fin design outperformed the NACA0012 design, generating more consistent thrust than the NACA profiled fin [17].

To fully emulate the motion of a tuna-like caudal fin (Figure 7.4) a robotic fin must not only be rotated but also moved from side to side (or up and down) in heave. Researchers at the Massachusetts Institute of Technology (MIT) have investigated how these two motions can be combined to produce forward thrust using a towed finning NACA0012-shaped hydrofoil [13,18]. For motion at very low Strouhal numbers the foil produced drag but as the Strouhal number was increased a thrust was produced. Experiments with this device confirmed that the Strouhal number range for good efficiency matched Strouhal numbers measured for fish and aquatic mammals. The best efficiency of 70% was obtained for $St = 0.25$ and a maximum angle of attack of 15°. They also showed that biasing the pitch angle on the moving foil can be a useful tool for maneuvering [18].

A tuna-like robot [19] has enabled MIT researchers to study the role of the body and tail in steady fish-like swimming. The robot, the shape of a Bluefin tuna, was towed while six electric motors pulling on internal cables caused the Lycra covered body to flex at six joints in a realistic way. The device has been used to measure the capacity for drag reduction by the active swimming body.

This measurement presents a challenge because the propulsor is also the body of the fish. To get around this obstacle two metrics for drag reduction detection were developed, one of which compared an "upper-bound" estimate of the drag force on the actively swimming robotic fish body to the drag encountered while towing the rigid robot body at the same speed [19]. Their study confirmed that active swimming involving body and tail results in real drag reduction. The flow was characterized by "body-bound vortices" shed at the tail into a propulsive wake. They suggested that swimming action promoted a laminar boundary layer while at the same time suppressing separation of the boundary layer, to form a wake. It is clear that for the fish, the body is part of the swimming mechanism and can play a major role in drag management.

The motion of water alongside a fish that is swimming in a flume can be studied by seeding the water with tiny reflective particles and then imaging particle displacements using laser or stroboscopic light to highlight position. Researchers at Woods Hole Oceanographic Institute have used this technique, known as digital particle image velocimetry (DPIV), to study the boundary layer in scup (*Stenotomus chrysops,* a small Atlantic Ocean carangiform swimmer) and

---

* The NACA0012 foil is symmetric with its maximum width 12% of chord length.

smooth dogfish (*Mustelus canis*, an anguilliform swimmer) [20]. Their results have shown that friction "skin" drag goes up when swimming, but that fish can delay or even eliminate boundary layer separation (see Chapter 6) and this should reduce form drag. How they do this must require careful tracking of water movements/pressures along the body.

It is becoming clear that fish can not only manipulate the vortices they create but also the vortices they encounter thereby affecting the load distribution on the body" [21]. For example, fish use vortices shed by the body and side fins by constructively combining them with tail vortices for enhancement of propulsion [21].

And it is through the generation of vortices, largely developed by the body during the "C shape" maneuver, that a fish can turn rapidly [12]. The "C shape" maneuver depicted in Figure 7.6 has been emulated in a soft fish-like robot with fully self-contained power and control of muscle-like devices by researchers at MIT [22]. The robot has a thin sheet-like "backbone" that can bend easily but is also stiff in-plane and is flanked on each side by hollow silicone devices that act like muscles. When the hollow chambers on one side are filled with a fluid under pressure (CO_2 in this case) they expand and this causes the entire tail to bend around.

Reef fish spend much of their time near and under archways and around rocks in moving water; places where you would never place a boat hull or large submersible. They can avoid collisions through feeling the water [23] and they can position themselves to harvest lift by sitting in the lee of vortices shed by upstream bodies. Trout can, in effect, surf these vortices, tuning their swimming to gain lift from the eddies shed in a steady flow [24]. While doing this, they adopt a unique pattern of body motion: termed the "Karman gait." Optimal positioning includes sitting in front of the cylinder, or in the bow wake; using their bodies, like a sail, to tack forward against the flow.

In order to sense the flow fields around them, fish use a sensory system called the lateral line (Figure 7.7). The basic sensor elements are "hair cells" very similar to the sensors in our inner ear. On the surface of the fish, these clusters of hair cells project

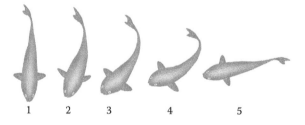

Figure 7.6 The C-shaped fish turning maneuver. (After Triantafyllou, M.S., Triantafyllou, G.S., and Yue, D.K.P. *Annual Review of Fluid Mechanics*, 32(1), 33–53, 2000 [12].) (Redrawn by Vivian L. Ward.)

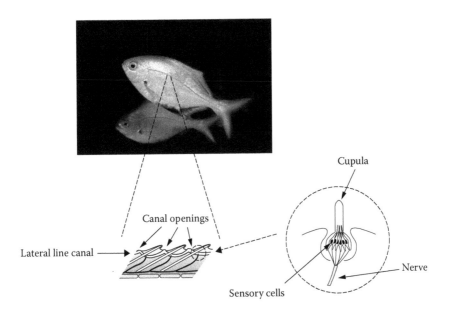

Figure 7.7 The principal transducer of the lateral line is the neuromast that consists of a group of hair cells with their microvilli projecting into a jelly-like cup (cupula). Some neuromasts project their cupula above the surface of the skin. Movement of water causes the cupula to bend and this entrains the cilia that translate the bending into the sensory stimulus. Other neuromasts, with modified cupulas are located beneath the surface in canals that run longitudinally along the fish. This group acts as transducers of the pressure gradient. (Redrawn by Vivian L. Ward.)

into the boundary layer and measure flow velocity, or are embedded in canals and detect the pressure difference between the canal openings. Some fish, such as cave dwelling species, have no eyes, and the lateral line provides their major spatial sense. As they glide through the water they create a flow field around the body that is sensed by the lateral line [23]. Obstacles in the water around the fish distort the flow field, and these distortions are sensed by the lateral line system. The term given to this ability is hydrodynamic imaging. Experiments manipulating different components of the lateral line system show that this sensory input is important in maintaining swimming efficiency in both steady and turbulent flows, in addition to providing important information allowing fish to orient toward prey and predators.

Although hydrodynamic imaging is very short range, a synthetic lateral line could provide a collision avoidance system for an autonomous unmanned vehicle.

A number of approaches have been used to generate artificial lateral line sensors and sensor arrays and these arrays have been successfully used to evaluate distance to source [25]. Engineers from Northwestern University have developed an artificial lateral line using MEMS (microelectromechanical system) technology that can accurately localize a vibrating source [26].

The fins of fish and their associated nerves might provide the ability to augment the flow sensing function of the lateral line. Consider the structure and function of the "bony" fish fin. Unlike the thick fins on the shark, the fins of teleosts (bony fish), are thin with bony rays that support the fin and act like spindly little fingers to move segments of a fin independently (Figure 7.8). A single fin ray is a composite structure consisting of bony columns or hemitrichs that are semicircular in cross section and separated by a fin membrane and other connective tissues. The base of each fin ray where it meets the fish's body sits atop a cartilage pad. Ligaments at the hemitrich bases are attached to tendons. Muscles that pull on these tendons cause one hemitrich to slide relative to the other so that the ray assumes a bent shape. The operation of an entire group of rays enables the fish to open the fin wide or close and fold it alongside the body or to create a rippling effect along the fin. A study of the neural activity of nerve fibers associated with fin rays (for the bluegill sunfish pectoral fins), suggests that finned fish can sense fin bending and position; valuable feedback for their control that is akin to proprioception [27], the ability to know position through in-built strain sensing. The strain sensors in our own musculature enables us to touch our nose with eyes closed. Perhaps this provides a mechanism for flow

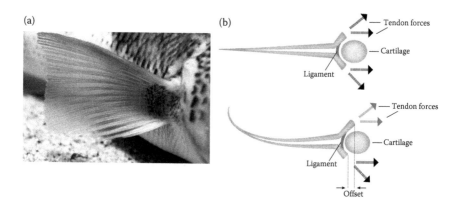

Figure 7.8 (a) The pectoral fin of a New Zealand blue cod (*Parapercis colias*). The fin rays are clearly visible in the photograph. (Photo by Iain A. Anderson.) (b) Each fin ray consists of two semicircular columns of bone (hemitrichs). A muscle set tugs at tendons that are attached to a ligament at the base of one of the hemitrichs. Pulling the hemitrich toward the base results in a smooth bending of the entire structure. (After Alben, S., Madden, P.G., and Lauder, G.V. *Journal of the Royal Society Interface*, 4(13), 243–256, 2007 [28].) (Redrawn by Vivian L. Ward. Photo by Iain A. Anderson.)

control so that fish feel the vortices they produce through their fins and activate their muscles appropriately.

Multiple fin ray operation has been investigated by researchers at Harvard who developed a model of the bluegill sunfish's pectoral fin [29]. The robotic fin with its separate motorized rays that emulate the fin rays of the sunfish pectoral has drawn attention to the need to research how to interpret sensory data from a robotic fin. Further breakthroughs would lead to the construction of control surfaces for a swimming robot using devices that both actuate, and self-sense [30]. It would then be possible for engineered finning devices to feel and respond to fluid vortices.

A biorobot or fish-like submersible could one day employ actuators that operate directly on body and fin control surfaces like natural muscles do. For example, one group at Wollongong has used ionic polymeric (polyppyrole) artificial muscles for this. The small robot that supported a camera provided a true fish-eye view and illustrated the use of a small finning robot as a means for inspection [31]. Electronic artificial muscles could also be employed. Their use for fish-swimming has already been demonstrated in the air: researchers at EMPA in Switzerland have built an 8 m long airship with artificial muscle actuators, made of dielectric elastomer, integrated with the skin enabling it to move like a fish [32] (Figure 7.9). These actuators are multifunctional [33] and could ultimately

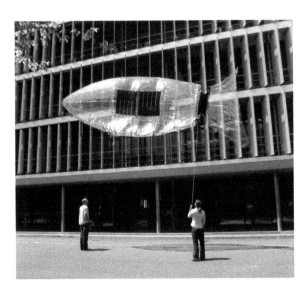

Figure 7.9 The EMPA fish-like blimp. Electroactive polymer actuators (dielectric elastomers) were used in the skin at the middle and at the joint between the tail and body. (Photo courtesy of Silvain Michel, EMPA.)

be used to emulate the inherent compliance, tunable stiffness, and self-sensing capabilities of natural muscle.

Therefore, it is now feasible for us to produce biomimetic fins with artificial muscle actuators that are orchestrated to move in a realistic way. But we face the near impossible task of coordinating movement between fins and body. And how can we get our actuators to respond to information from the water surrounding them? Again we look to fish for a solution. The athleticism and maneuverability that we see in these top ocean predators was enabled by an innovation, not in the "hardware" of fins and muscles, but in the "software" of brain structures and circuits.

Fish are chordates, the group to which we ourselves belong. The earliest chordates were worm-like, but running along the length of the body they had a notochord, essentially a flexible rod that resists shortening. On either side of the rod were segmented muscle blocks. With this simple arrangement, a wave of muscle activity alternating down the two sides of the body could produce undulation and propel the animal forward. Early in chordate evolution the notochord was supplanted by the vertebral column, which has retained its basic form and function from the earliest jawless vertebrates (hagfish and lampreys) through to ourselves. Like modern fishes, hagfish (Figure 7.10) and lampreys swim with body undulations. But they have little in the way of a tail fin, and they lack the paired fins that play such an important role in the control of swimming in most fishes. The first vertebrates to have jaws were the elasmobranchs whose living representatives include sharks, skates, and rays. Along with the advent of jaws, early elasmobranchs had a distinct tail fin, and the two sets of paired fins (pectoral and pelvic fins). The paired fins not only play a key role in the control of locomotion, but have also proved to be a versatile basis for the eventual evolution of legs, arms, and wings!

Hagfish and lampreys have the basic vertebrate plan of three major brain compartments (Figure 7.10): the forebrain, midbrain, and hindbrain. Each of those compartments is associated with a major sensory system; olfaction with the forebrain, vision with the midbrain, and balance and hearing with the hindbrain. But there is one brain compartment that sharks and we as jawed vertebrates have that is missing from our jawless ancestors. This is the cerebellum, which in humans account for well over half the nerve cells in the brain! The cerebellum appeared at the same time as jaws and paired fins, and it is a reasonable claim that it formed part of an innovation package that carried with it the potential for the command of 3D environments that we see in today's fishes, birds, and mammals.

The cerebellum then is an "add-on" compartment to the brain, added over the top of existing motor circuits and reflexes. This is paralleled by the layered subsumption architecture in robotic [34] and complex computing systems where overlying layers are increasingly abstract, but subsume the simpler underlying

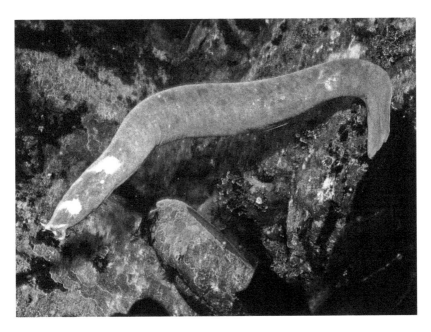

Figure 7.10 The New Zealand hagfish (*Eptatretus cirrhatus*) that lacks eyes, a jaw, and paired fins; it feeds by sucking onto its prey with its circular mouth and then stabbing and rasping through the flesh with a tooth-studded tongue. (Photo by Malcolm Francis.)

ones [24,25]; in the sense that each higher layer provides constraints on the "valid" behaviors in the layer beneath it, through inhibition or the suppression of operations [34] (Figure 7.11). Although for the biological sense this may be implemented somewhat differently one of the best-documented roles of the cerebellum is its ability to implement gain control on the open loop reflexes that stabilize the eyes during head movement. In this case, error in the reflex induces learning in the cerebellum that corrects the gain on the reflex pathway. Subsequently, the learning is transferred to the direct reflex pathway. So in this version of subsumption architecture the cerebellum level is not normally directly involved in the lower level reflex, but can intervene in the reflex pathway if required, and may even supervise corrective adjustments in the lower level.

Current work is more focused on understanding how the cerebellum works [35,36], rather than trying to mimic it in a machine, but once we understand it there will be substantial rewards.

If the cerebellum exerts a control layer over the top of existing brain circuits, what is the core functionality of the cerebellar circuitry that supports this?

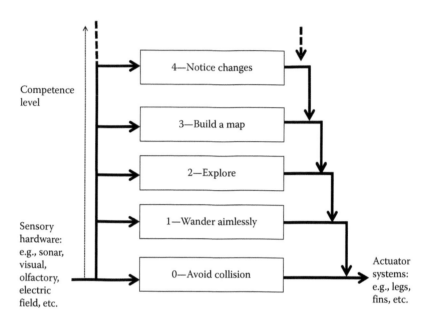

Figure 7.11 A schematic of the subsumption architecture described by Rodney Brooks in the 1980s, for the control of a mobile robot, in a paper cited more than 9000 times [34]! The architecture allows for a system to be enhanced by simply adding higher levels of competence to an existing function. Each competence level, "an informal specification for a set of behaviors" builds upon a working system whose sublayers operate reliably and robustly. In this example, the most basic competence level for a mobile robot involves the avoidance of collision. This first layer operates reliably and is not altered. A new layer can now be added (1) to enable aimless wander around without bumping into other objects. Above this, a layer of control enables the robot to (2) explore its world by moving toward and identifying nearby objects. From its experience, the robot can build a map (3). The further ability to identify changes in the world (4) can now follow. Each higher layer provides constraints on the "valid" behaviors in the layer beneath it, through inhibition or the suppression of operations. In the biological case of the cerebellum the subsumption definition of adding higher levels of competence to an existing function still applies but in a different sense as described in the text. (After Brooks, R.A. *A Robust Layered Control System for a Mobile Robot.* 1985, Massachusetts Institute of Technology [34].) (Drawing by Iain A. Anderson.)

It is currently viewed like a computer chip: the "cerebellar chip" that is a circuit module that can meet multiple control needs. Identifying the function of a particular cerebellar chip requires knowledge of both the chip's algorithm and its individual connections. The lead "candidate algorithm" is an adaptive filter (Figure 7.12). One use of an adaptive filter is to identify the noise component of

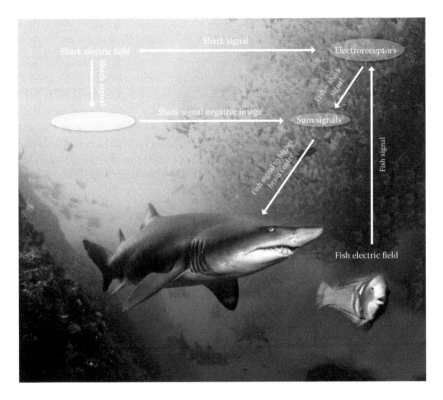

Figure 7.12 The signal that is sensed by the electrosensors on the shark comes from the field created by the fish plus the background noise of the shark. A cerebellum-like structure in the shark's brain performs the role of an adaptive filter finding the correct negative image for the shark's own background noise. When combined with the signal, the noise is removed, revealing the electric field for the fish. (Drawing and photos by Iain A. Anderson.)

an input signal and then use the inverse of the noisy component (mirror image) to cancel it from the original input signal [37]. The adaptive filter algorithm is "computationally powerful" enough to be used in a very wide variety of engineering applications.

To better understand the idea of the cerebellar chip as an adaptive filter, we again turn to the evolutionary origins of the cerebellum. The precursor to the cerebellum was a cerebellum-like structure found in the hindbrain of jawless vertebrates and also in sharks and their close relatives. Lampreys and hagfish have cerebellum-like parts of the brain, whereas sharks and other fish have the cerebellum-like structures along with a true cerebellum. The cerebellum-like structure qualifies, both in terms of its wiring, and its function, as an early model of the cerebellar chip. In this case, the chip is plugged into the direct sensory pathways of flow sensing and electrosensory systems. Without going into any detail about these sensory systems, the one thing we need to know is that both systems are prone to the problem of self-generated noise.

Consider, for example, the electrosensory system of the shark (refer to Chapter 9): Sharks detect the weak electric fields of their prey, but also generate similar fields themselves. In both systems, the cerebellum chip solves the self-generated noise problem. It provides an adaptive filter that creates a negative image of the self-generated noise allowing it to be canceled before the information is sent to higher brain centers. In effect, the cerebellum-like structure is the biological equivalent of noise canceling headphones. In this case, biology has beaten our own technology by a mere 400 million years or so.

There may be other biomimetic innovations derived from the cerebellar chip in the areas of swimming efficiency and control. One possible use of the chip may be in adaptive control of boundary layer flow. This was discussed earlier as a means for drag reduction: Direct measurement of the boundary layer in a freely swimming fish shows that fish can actively avoid boundary layer separation [20]. And this is highly advantageous for drag reduction for when the boundary layer that surrounds the immersed body separates from the body, a broad wake is created that is filled with turbulent vortices (refer to Chapter 6). Avoiding this must involve both sensing and closely controlled activation of fins and body. At this point it is not known how, or even if, the cerebellum is directly involved in active boundary layer control. However, there is direct evidence for a role of flow sensing in swimming efficiency [38] and the cerebellum certainly provides a candidate mechanism for an error minimizing adaptive filter, which could help tune swimming motion.

The cerebellum is also likely to be involved in the delicate postural control necessary for fish with swim bladders. This is due to their inherent roll instability (Chapter 5). It is almost certainly involved in the control of fins for everything from swimming to prey capture and all the other day-to-day activities of fish. Stability, control, and efficiency will all be key performance attributes of soft robots underwater. Although our current understanding of the cerebellum does not provide us with device-ready biomimetic control, the attempt to implement cerebellar-like control will be an important test of how well we understand biological systems and how effectively we can mimic them. Undoubtedly, the positive feedback between the biological research on the adaptive control of movement and the technological implementation of biomimetic technologies will enhance both our understanding of biology and its real-world biomimetic applications.

Future work must focus on the incorporation of machine learning techniques for training biomimetic fin-like propulsors. If we persist, we may one day see robotic finned propulsors on fish-like bodies on the surface of the sea and

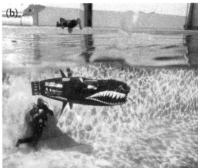

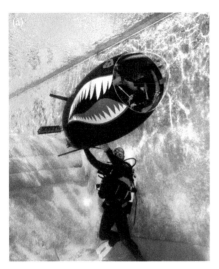

Figure 7.13 (a) A front view of the fin-propelled, human-powered racing submarine (*Taniwha*, Biomimetics Lab Auckland Bioengineering Institute), that competed at the 13th International Submarine Races held in Carderock, Maryland, June 22–26, 2015. (b) The submarine is propelled by a diver that pedals two *Hobie Mirage* fin drives fitted to ventral and dorsal surfaces. This was the fastest nonpropeller submarine at these races, achieving a speed of 3.65 knots (1.88 m/s), that compared well with the best of the propeller-driven human submarines. (Photos by Iain A. Anderson.)

beneath it that can sense their own movements and process the data using something akin to a cerebellar chip. Such fin-powered devices could well support humans too (Figure 7.13) extending our ability to explore the underwater world. And when this happens the fin may well finally upstage the screw propeller.

References

1. Wardle, C.S., Videler, J.J., Arimoto, T., Franco, J.M., and He, P. The muscle twitch and the maximum swimming speed of giant bluefin tuna, *Thunnus thynnus* L. *Journal of Fish Biology*, 1989. 35(1): 129–137.
2. Fish, F.E. Power output and propulsive efficiency of swimming bottlenose dolphins (*Tursiops truncatus*). *Journal of Experimental Biology*, 1993. 185(1): 179–193.
3. Fish, F.E. and Rohr, J.J. *Review of Dolphin Hydrodynamics and Swimming Performance.* 1999, U.S. Navy Technical Report 1801, SPAWAR Systems Center San Diego.
4. Joubert, P. *Some Aspects of Submarine Design Part 1. Hydrodynamics.* 2004, Victoria, Australia: Australian Defense Science and Technology Organisation.

5. Colman, J.G. A review of the biology and ecology of the whale shark. *Journal of Fish Biology*, 1997. 51(6): 1219–1234.
6. Vogel, S. *Life in Moving Fluids: The Physical Biology of Flow.* 1994, Princeton, NJ: Princeton University Press.
7. Breslin, J.P. and Andersen, P. *Hydrodynamics of Ship Propellers.* Cambridge Ocean Technology, Series 3. 1994, Cambridge, UK: Cambridge University Press. 559pp.
8. Jones, F.R.H. Tail beat frequency, amplitude, and swimming speed of a shark tracked by sector scanning sonar. *Journal du Conseil*, 1973. 35(1): 95–97.
9. Webb, P.W., Kostecki, P.T., and Stevens, E.D. The effect of size and swimming speed on locomotor kinematics of rainbow trout. *Journal of Experimental Biology*, 1984. 109(1): 77–95.
10. Bainbridge, R. The speed of swimming of fish as related to size and to the frequency and amplitude of the tail beat. *Journal of Experimental Biology*, 1958. 35(1): 109–133.
11. Sfakiotakis, M., Lane, D.M., and Davies, J.B.C. Review of fish swimming modes for aquatic locomotion. *IEEE Journal of Oceanic Engineering*, 1999. 24(2).
12. Triantafyllou, M.S., Triantafyllou, G.S., and Yue, D.K.P. Hydrodynamics of fishlike swimming. *Annual Review of Fluid Mechanics*, 2000. 32(1): 33–53.
13. Triantafyllou, G.S., Triantafyllou, M.S., and Grosenbaugh, M.A. Optimal thrust development in oscillating foils with application to fish propulsion. *Journal of Fluids and Structures*, 1993. 7(2): 205–224.
14. Fish, F.E., Weber, P.W., Murray, M.M., and Howle, L.E. The tubercles on humpback whales' flippers: Application of bio-inspired technology. *Integrative and Comparative Biology*, 2011. 51(1): 203–213.
15. Miklosovic, D.S., Murray, M.M., Howle, L.E., and Fish, F.E. Leading-edge tubercles delay stall on humpback whale (*Megaptera novaeangliae*) flippers. *Physics of Fluids*, 2004. 16(5): L39–L42.
16. Weihs, D. Stability versus maneuverability in aquatic locomotion. *Integrative and Comparative Biology*, 2002. 42(1): 127–134.
17. Riggs, P., Bowyer, A., and Vincent, J. Advantages of a biomimetic stiffness profile in pitching flexible fin propulsion. *Journal of Bionic Engineering*, 2010. 7(2): 113–119.
18. Schouveiler, L., Hover, F.S., and Triantafyllou, M.S. Performance of flapping foil propulsion. *Journal of Fluids and Structures*, 2005. 20(7 Special issue): 949–959.
19. Barrett, D.S., Triantafyllou, M.S., Yue, D.K.P., Grosenbaugh, M.A., and Wolfgang, M.J. Drag reduction in fish-like locomotion. *Journal of Fluid Mechanics*, 1999. 392(1): 183–212.
20. Anderson, E.J., McGillis, W.R., and Grosenbaugh, M.A. The boundary layer of swimming fish. *Journal of Experimental Biology*, 2001. 204(1): 81–102.
21. Zhu, Q., Wolfgang, M.J., Yue, D.K.P., and Triantafyllou, M.S. Three-dimensional flow structures and vorticity control in fish-like swimming. *Journal of Fluid Mechanics*, 2002. 468: 1–28.
22. Marchese, A.D., Onal, C.D., and Rus, D. Autonomous soft robotic fish capable of escape maneuvers using fluidic elastomer actuators. *Soft Robotics*, 2014. 1(1): 75–87.
23. Windsor, S.P., Norris, S.E., Cameron, S.M., Mallinson, G.D., and Montgomery, J.C. The flow fields involved in hydrodynamic imaging by blind Mexican cave fish (*Astyanax fasciatus*). Part I: Open water and heading towards a wall. *Journal of Experimental Biology*, 2010. 213(22): 3819–3831.
24. Liao, J.C., Beal, D.N., Lauder, G.V., and Triantafyllou, M.S. The Karman gait: Novel body kinematics of rainbow trout swimming in a vortex street. *Journal of Experimental Biology*, 2003. 206(6): 1059–1073.
25. Dagamseh, A., Wiegerink, R., Lammerink, T., and Krijnen, G. Imaging dipole flow sources using an artificial lateral-line system made of biomimetic hair flow sensors. *Journal of the Royal Society Interface*, 2013. 10(83).

114

26. Yang, Y., Nguyen, N., Chen, N., Lockwood, M., Tucker, C., Hu, H., Bleckmann, H., Liu, C., and Jones, D.L. Artificial lateral line with biomimetic neuromasts to emulate fish sensing. *Bioinspiration & Biomimetics*, 2010. 5(1): 016001.
27. Williams IV, R., Neubarth, N., and Hale, M.E. The function of fin rays as proprioceptive sensors in fish. *Nature Communications*, 2013. 4: 1729.
28. Alben, S., Madden, P.G., and Lauder, G.V. The mechanics of active fin-shape control in ray-finned fishes. *Journal of the Royal Society Interface*, 2007. 4(13): 243–256.
29. Phelan, C., Tangorra, J., Lauder, G., and Hale, M. A biorobotic model of the sunfish pectoral fin for investigations of fin sensorimotor control. *Bioinspiration & Biomimetics*, 2010. 5(3).
30. Bandyopadhyay, P.R. Trends in biorobotic autonomous undersea vehicles. *IEEE Journal of Oceanic Engineering*, 2005. 30(1): 109–139.
31. McGovern, S., Alici, G., Truong, V-T., and Spinks, G. Finding NEMO (novel electro-material muscle oscillator): A polypyrrole powered robotic fish with real-time wireless speed and directional control. *Smart Materials and Structures*, 2009. 18(9): 095009.
32. Jordi, C., Michel, S., and Fink, E. Fish-like propulsion of an airship with planar membrane dielectric elastomer actuators. *Bioinspiration & Biomimetics*, 2010. 5(2): 026007.
33. Anderson, I.A., Gisby, T.A., McKay, T.G., O'Brien, B.M., and Calius, E.P. Multi-functional dielectric elastomer artificial muscles for soft and smart machines. *Journal of Applied Physics*, 2012. 112(4): 041101.
34. Brooks, R.A. *A Robust Layered Control System for a Mobile Robot*. 1985, Massachusetts Institute of Technology.
35. Montgomery, J.C., Bodznick, D.A., and Yopak, K.E. The cerebellum and cerebellum-like structures of cartilaginous fishes. *Brain Behavior and Evolution*, 2012. 80: 152–165.
36. Yopak, K.E., Lisney, T.J., Darlington, R.B., Collin, S.P., Montgomery, J.C., and Finlay, B.L. A conserved pattern of brain scaling from sharks to primates. *Proceedings of the National Academy of Sciences*, 2010. 107(29): 12946–12951.
37. Porrill, J., Dean, P., and Anderson, S.R. Adaptive filters and internal models: Multilevel description of cerebellar function. *Neural Networks*, 2013. 47: 134–149.
38. Yanase, K., Herbert, N.A., and Montgomery, J.C. Disrupted flow sensing impairs hydro-dynamic performance and increases the metabolic cost of swimming in the yellowtail kingfish, *Seriola lalandi. Journal of Experimental Biology*, 2012. 215(22): 3944–3954.

Chapter 8 Listening to the silent world

The sound of an outboard motor can put a diver into a state of high alert, aware that a trip back to the surface is fraught with the danger of being struck by a boat. It is impossible for us to judge the direction, or distance to a sound source underwater: the normal cues we use to localize sound in air simply do not work underwater. In addition, much of the sound we hear is from the operation of our own demand regulator. Holding our breath to listen raises the risk of lung embolism if we are ascending. But if we safely stop and listen we can hear the sounds of breaking waves, boat propellers, grunting and chewing fish, snapping shrimps, whale song, and dolphin calls. For the creatures that inhabit the sea, these sounds are ideal for communication and navigation.

Compared with light that is heavily absorbed and scattered by seawater, limiting visibility to tens of meters, and chemical scents that are dispersed by ocean currents, sound is an effective medium for underwater information transfer. Sound can travel long distances, and propagates in all directions. For instance, the sound intensity (power/unit area) of a wave of frequency 500 Hz, in the middle of the hearing range of many fish, will drop by about 1 decibel* (dB), about 20%, over 100 km due to attenuation by seawater alone [1]. Of course, sound intensity will also be affected by the geometry of propagation, as it radiates away from a point source such as a singing whale.

For whales, lower frequencies that are much less attenuated by seawater are particularly favorable for long-distance communication. Among the sound repertoire of the fin whale is a 1 s downward frequency sweep from 25 to 15 Hz, referred to as a chirp [2]. It is believed that this sound can put it into contact with other whales hundreds of kilometers away [3].

Acoustic communication over such long distances presents an interesting physical challenge. The ocean is on average about 4.5 km deep, so for a sound wave to travel hundreds of kilometers would require for it to be guided, keeping it in mid-water and minimizing energy loss associated with reflection off the surface or sea bottom. The Sound Fixing and Ranging (SOFAR) channel or Deep Sound

---

* The number of dB (decibels) represents 10 times the logarithm to base 10 of the ratio of two power quantities. A power ratio of 10 times would be 10 dB and a power ratio of 100 times would be 20 dB.

Channel, discovered in the 1940s, is a deepwater waveguide for sound exploited by marine creatures such as the fin whale [3] and submarines. It works on the relationship between sound speed and depth. Sound travels faster near the surface where temperature is relatively high. As depth increases so temperature drops and temperature drop is accompanied by a slowing of sound speed. Pressure increases with depth and this has the opposite effect on sound speed, increasing it. At a depth that is of the order of hundreds of meters the sound speed profile passes through a minimum. This defines the axis of the SOFAR channel. A sound wave that deviates from the axis of the SOFAR channel will be refracted back toward it by the faster sonic speeds near the surface and at depth.

Any acoustic information, whether from fish, marine mammal, or man, must be discerned against the background noise in the sea that comes from many natural and man-made sources (Figure 8.1). Wind-driven waves produce sound at low frequencies (~10 Hz) through to high frequencies (~25 kHz) that are outside our range of hearing. Watercraft can generate sounds at low frequencies in the tens of Hertz (large ships) and at kilohertz frequencies (small propeller-driven pleasure craft). Over the past few decades, human noise associated with commercial and recreation boating, military and civilian SONARs, and oil exploration, has led

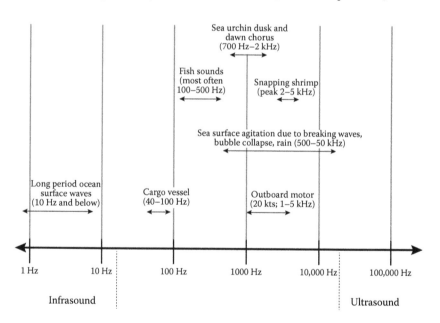

Figure 8.1 Typical frequency ranges for some ambient noise sources in the ocean. (From the review by Hildebrand, J.A. *Marine Ecology Progress Series*, 395, 5–20, 2009 [6].) (Sea urchin data are from Radford, C., Jeffs, A., Tindle, C., and Montgomery, J.C. *Marine Ecology Progress Series*, 362, 37–43, 2008 [7].)

to an increase in overall background noise level of about 12 dB [4]; a 16 times increase! There is concern that the mating songs of the large male baleen whales, such as the fin whale, might be obscured by these rising levels of human noise [5].

Shallow reefs are very noisy places, due largely to grazing animals, snapping shrimps, and vocalizing fish. For instance, at dawn and dusk along the shallow reefs around New Zealand there is a noisy chorus of scraping sounds when kina (*Evechinus chloroticus*), a local species of sea urchin, come out of their daytime cavities to feed. Each urchin that grazes rock for algae produces a resonant vibration of the fluid within the hemispherical chamber of its own skeleton. This is a "Helmholtz" cavity resonance largely determined by the volume enclosed by the skeleton and the area at the opening of the urchin's mouth. A Helmholtz cavity resonance is excited when blowing across the top of an empty bottle. And like the bottle, size matters: larger bottles/urchins generate lower frequency tones. It is likely that much of the New Zealand reef noise at dusk and dawn comes from urchins producing a background of noise at frequencies between 700 and 2000 Hz [7]. Surface grazing fish contribute to this noise, such as the Red moki (*Cheilodactylus spectabilis*) that bump against, and take small bites from, the rocky reef, turning much of the pulverized material into sand that is flushed backward and out of its gills.

Vocalizing reef fish also contribute to this sound milieu, advertising their presence to a possible mate, warning off intruders, and maintaining contact with others in the group. The noises they make are described in the scientific literature as grunts, growls, purrs, croaks, pops, and squawks. There are two main mechanism for producing these sounds: the rubbing together of body parts (stridulation) such as the grinding of teeth or plucking fin ray tendons and vibrations of their gas-filled swim bladder. Some tropical triggerfish can produce sounds from their swim bladder by beating their body like a drum with their pectoral fins. Other fish use sonic muscles that are attached directly to the swim bladder. For example, a small nocturnal fish that lives in caves along the reefs of New Zealand, the Bigeye (*Pempheris adspersa*), uses two sonic muscles that are attached directly to its swim bladder to produce popping sounds that are quite audible to the diver. At night they leave their caves and rocky crevasses to forage near the reef and in the dark perhaps using the popping sound to maintain contact with others in the group [8]. Reef sounds play an important role in the recruitment of new reef residents from the larval fish and crustaceans that drift past the reef with the plankton. The noises provide navigational cues that enable them to find the reef and take up residence there [9].

For humans, the use of sound for underwater navigation is not feasible because we lose all of our ability to localize sound direction. Hearing sensitivity is lost too although compared with some fishes and marine mammals we are doing well at frequencies in the kilohertz range (Figure 8.2) [10]. To identify ways of improving

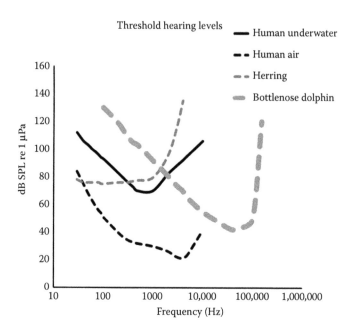

Figure 8.2 Comparison of threshold hearing levels for human hearing in air and underwater. (Original data were sound pressure level, SPL, relative to 20 μPa. This has been rescaled for SPL relative to 1 μPa.) (From Parvin, S.J. and Nedwell, J.R. *Underwater Technology: The International Journal of the Society for Underwater*, 21(1), 12–19, 1995 [10].) The Herring (*Clupea harengus*), which is based on composite data from the same author collected for several fish. (From Enger, P.S. *Comparative Biochemistry and Physiology*, 22(2), 527–538, 1967 [11].) The bottlenose dolphin—original data recorded from several dolphins have been encapsulated into a general trend-line here. (From Johnson, S.C. *Marine Bio-Acoustic*, W. Talvoga, Editor. 1967, New York, NY: Pergamon Press. pp. 247–260 [12].)

hearing sensitivity and our ability to judge sound direction we start by considering how our normal hearing mechanism operates in air and how this is affected by immersion in water.

The hearing mechanism of humans and other terrestrial vertebrates is configured to work in a relatively low noise environment. Much of what we hear comes from weak pressure fluctuations of airborne sound that are channeled onto the eardrum by each ear pinna (the external flap that is the visible part of our ear) and the ear canal (Figure 8.3). The ear canal can do this because it is lined with living tissue that has higher characteristic acoustic impedance than air. By this we mean that its tissue has a greater resistance to the flow of sound vibrations through it than air. Materials can be compared using impedance, which is simply the wave speed in the material multiplied by its density. If there is a big difference

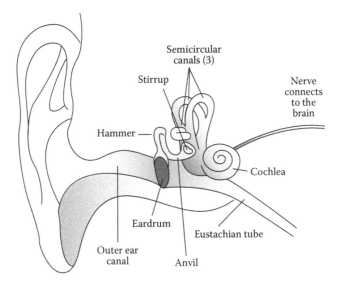

Figure 8.3 Human hearing mechanism and schematic illustrating the mechanical linkage from the outer ear to the inner ear. In addition to sensing sound, our hearing mechanism provides a sense of angular and linear accelerations, including gravity. The semicircular canals and otolith organs of the inner ear provide us with our sense of head rotation, with one semicircular canal for each of three orthogonal planes. These elements of the inner ear make up what is called the vestibular system. (Drawing by Vivian L. Ward.)

between the acoustic impedances of two materials then sound will be either reflected or absorbed. If the two impedances are the same then sound will pass through unhindered. The characteristic acoustic impedances of the tissue lining the ear and air are about 1.6×10^6 and 400 kg/m^2 s, respectively. The ratio of the two impedances is about 4000. A consequence of this huge impedance mismatch between the two is that the walls of the tissue-lined ear canal will not allow sound to pass through but instead will reflect the sound toward the eardrum, as it should.

The eardrum and bony linkages of the middle ear transmit vibrations into the liquid-filled cochlea of the inner ear. Vibratory motion of membranes within the cochlea provide a graded continuum of frequency-selective channels covering the range of our hearing from approximately 20 Hz to 20 kHz. The motions of the membranes displace cilia bundles that project from exquisitely sensitive displacement sensors, the hair cells. The sensory cells connect to the brain by nerve fibers.

When we are submerged in the sea our ear canal, filled with water, is ineffective at channeling sound to the eardrum. The characteristic acoustic impedance of its tissue is similar to that of water (about 1.5×10^6 kg/m^2 s), therefore sound will pass through it instead of being reflected from its walls. Bone's characteristic impedance is only about 5 times greater than water and is also capable of absorbing sound from water, so that most of what we hear underwater is attributable to sound conduction through the bones of our skull to our inner ear. Although our hearing sensitivity is reduced, this mechanism serves us reasonably well for frequencies up to a couple of kilohertz (Figure 8.2).

We can hear sound underwater, but none of our usual mechanisms for determining sound direction work. One of them is related to the difference in arrival time of sound waves at each ear when the sound source is off-center (Figure 8.4). This is the interaural time difference. Given a typical diameter for the human head (say 20 cm) and the speed of sound in air (about 340 m/s at sea level) the maximum interaural time difference, when the sound is directly off to one side will be approximately 600 μs. As the source moves toward the midline, the difference will get smaller. Therefore, to effectively use interaural time differences we need to be able to discriminate arrival times of sound at our two ears by 30 μs or so

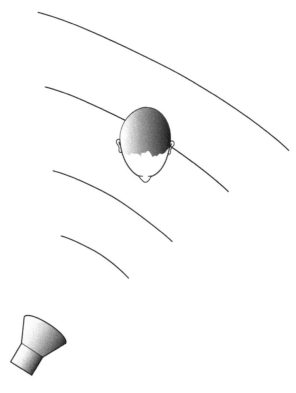

Figure 8.4 The interaural time difference is the time interval between a sound wave's arrival at both ears. Arriving at the right ear first in this drawing. (Drawing by Mark T. Ryan.)

(the time difference between the ears for a sound off the midline by about 3°), which we do! Physiological studies on other animals have shown that the brain uses the information contained in the arrival time of nerve-generated spikes [13]. The model for how this might work was described by Lloyd Jeffress of Caltech [14], and is now referred to as the neuronal delay-line comparator. The neuronal delay-line comparator turns a time-based event into spatial information that can be directly linked to the sound direction. With standard electronics the principle can be used for analog to digital signal conversion [15]. A schematic for a delay-line comparator is depicted in Figure 8.5.

The speed of sound is over 4 times faster in water than in air (~1500 m/s), requiring us to be able to discriminate much smaller time delays that lie beyond the capability of our own internal delay-line comparator. For this to function we would need to put our ears at least 4 times further apart when fully submerged: about 1 meter. Interestingly, mechanical pinna devices were built like this during WWI and the early part of WWII to determine the location of incoming enemy aircraft. The operator sat between the enormous metal pinnae.

A second mechanism for sound direction sensing is associated with the sound shadow provided by our head (Figure 8.6): the sound will be on the side that is louder to us. This is the interaural intensity difference. The effective sound shadow created by the head is frequency-dependent and better for higher frequencies when the wavelength is about the width of our head or smaller (>2 kHz in air). However, in water audible wavelengths are over 4 times longer so that the sound shadow provided by our head is virtually ineffective for direction sensing.

A third mechanism is spectral shaping: the direction-dependent altering of the frequency components of sound. In air this is provided by our external ears, or pinnae. Each pinna changes the character of sound coming from behind; acting as frequency-selective filters, making sources that come from behind sound dull in comparison with the same source located toward the front [16]. But our pinnae are of similar characteristic acoustic impedance to water, so they are completely ineffective at influencing the spectrum of the incoming underwater sound and the sound passes through them unchanged.

If our pinnae work better in air then why not surround them with air while underwater? This has been investigated by researchers in Israel using a face mask assembly (ProEar 2000) that keeps the ear canal dry by covering each pinna with a watertight silicone-sealed ear-pod [17]. Air is able to travel along tubing that connects each ear-pod with the mask and this enables the diver to maintain ambient pressure within each pod. One objective is to keep the ears dry, thus reducing the likelihood of ear infection.

The pure tone hearing thresholds of 10 healthy divers were evaluated in a tank; each wearing a ProEar mask and a standard mask. There was no significant

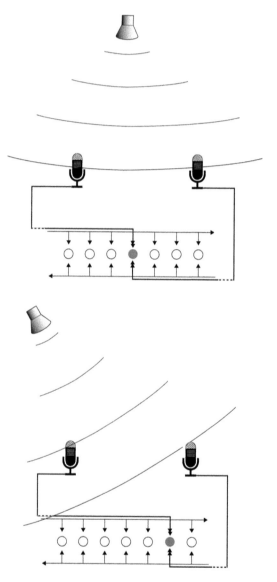

Figure 8.5 Delay line comparator for sound localization. At the top, the sound source is equidistant from both microphones. At the bottom, the sound target is off to the left, so the left microphone picks up the sound first, and that information is transmitted down the upper delay line. Sound arrives later at the right microphone, so it travels only a short distance down the lower delay line before these two signals meet. The comparator "artificial" neurons fire when they receive input from each delay line. In this way, the comparator artificial neurons help to compile a map of where the sound is located. (Drawing by Mark T. Ryan.)

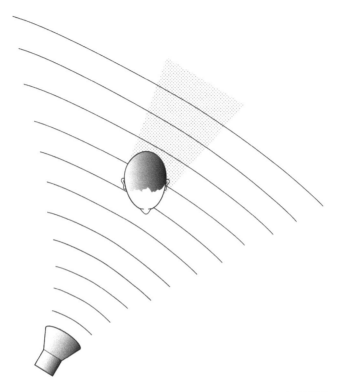

Figure 8.6 Interaural intensity difference. At higher frequencies (>2 kHz) our head will be effective at shadowing sound. In the drawing, the subject's left ear is in the sound shadow. (Drawing by Mark T. Ryan.)

improvement in hearing ability or in the ability to judge sound direction with the ProEar. The study concluded that the principal mode for human hearing underwater is through bone conduction.

Like us, toothed whales rely on bone for the conduction of sound from water to inner ear. We hear better than they do up to about 1 kHz or so, but at higher frequencies our hearing thresholds rise steeply, whereas theirs continue to improve, with the best sensitivity at tens of kilohertz, well above our range of hearing (Figure 8.2). For the bottlenose dolphin, the lower jawbone plays a key role in this. Within the jaw of the dolphin, there are at least four independent channels on each side filled with fat. These channels enlarge toward the rear of the jaw, improving the transfer of sound from water to bone and acting as waveguides [18,19]. And in the place of the thin and soft tympanic membrane of terrestrial mammals they have a large and thin tympanic bony plate. The dolphin's tympanic plate is 8 times larger than the human tympanic membrane. Together these two structures do a good job of explaining how the dolphin's acoustic sensitivity could exceed ours by a factor of 50–100 and may perhaps provide biomimetic design principals for devices that would augment our hearing abilities underwater.

Dolphin might use spectral shaping by the water itself: if the dolphin knows the source's sound then it will be able to judge the distance of the source not only from the drop-off in intensity of the sound with distance but also from the spectrum of the sound as higher frequencies will be attenuated more. Instead of external pinnae, that would be useless anyway and detract from swimming efficiency, they can also use the directionally dependent sound attenuating properties of their head. Structures within the head will more readily absorb higher frequencies and so the direction in which the head is pointing will influence the spectrum of the sound heard by the dolphin. For this to work well there are two conditions to be met: (1) the sound spectrum should be broad (not a monotone) so that it includes a range of frequencies that will each be attenuated differently by the head, (2) the frequencies should be relatively high [19], presumably so that their wavelengths are comparable or shorter than the head and can be selectively attenuated by it.

Dolphins and other toothed whales are fortunate in being able to control the frequency content of the sound they hear using their own high-frequency vocalizations for echolocation in the forward direction (Figure 8.7). Echolocation is the animal's form of active acoustics. The dolphin can produce a sound pulse broad enough in frequency that the range to the target can be accurately estimated due to spectral shaping by the water.

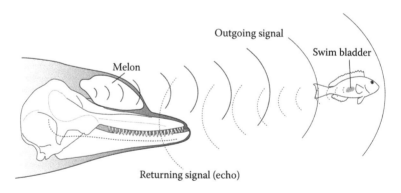

Figure 8.7 The dolphin clicking sound is produced by blowing air past the sonic lips behind the blowhole. The sonic lips are evolved from a nose-like structure. The air causes the lip membranes to vibrate and thus the clicking sound is produced. The sound passes through the melon that acts like an acoustic lens refracting the sound and directing it into a cone-shaped beam. The melon that contains a lipid material lies below the bump on the dolphin's forehead. The echo from the click, in this example, largely coming from reflections off the fish prey's swim bladder, is received by the lower jaw that acts as a waveguide. (Drawing by Vivian L. Ward.)

Our own form of active acoustics is referred to as SONAR (SOund NAvigation and Ranging), for which a pulse of sound emitted from a transmitter reflects from objects at a distance. The use of SONAR, for detecting icebergs, was put forward by Lewis Fry Richardson in a patent proposal that was filed soon after the sinking of the *Titanic*. The technology is now in everyday use by amateur fishers for fish finding.

Acoustic recording devices attached directly to toothed whales have revealed the details of echolocation interactions of these whales with their prey [20]. During their search for prey, the whales emit loud broadband clicks. As the whales close in on prey their emitted pulses are reduced in amplitude but produced more frequently so that they form a "buzz." Such lower intensity calls are less likely to alarm the prey, but due to the proximity of the prey still provide effective echoes. Because the return time of the echo is shortened by proximity, the time between echolocation clicks can be decreased by a corresponding amount, providing a substantially improved acoustic resolution of the target. In the same way that the bat's echolocation provided a biomimetic inspiration for radar, the details of how animals use active SONAR in the ocean may provide design considerations for our active acoustics applications.

For example, in situations where sediment or bubbles may incapacitate SONAR, dolphins are still able to use their echolocation. Indeed species such as the Atlantic bottlenose dolphin use bubble nets to corral their prey. This will also make it difficult for the dolphin to see their prey. Perhaps they solve this problem by exploiting the fact that clicks of different amplitude will scatter nonlinearly from the bubbles, meaning that the difference between the amplitude clicks emitted by the dolphin will not be the same as the difference between the signals that bounce back to the dolphin. With some neural processing it might be possible for the dolphin to separate the bubble reflections from the prey reflections [21].

Fish also have a sense that is analogous to echolocation. For this, they use their lateral line. But this operates at much lower frequencies and for sensing water movements at distances comparable to the length of the fish (refer to Chapter 7).

Fish hear well and vocalize at much lower frequencies than the toothed whales: from tens of Hertz up to a kilohertz. Their hearing mechanism is capable of localizing sound direction, but in a way very different to that of terrestrial animals, and aquatic mammals [9]. They too have hair cells that sense vibration; the hair cells of our cochlea are directly inherited from hair cell receptors found in the inner ear, and the lateral line organs of early fishes. The big differences came about because the wavelengths of audible sound are typically greater than the fish's body length. For example, the wavelength of sound in water at 1.5 kHz, a frequency above the sensitive range for many fish, is 1 m. One meter is substantially longer than most fish. Their tissue is also of a density similar to water and their characteristic acoustic impedance is about the same too. So as a sound wave passes a fish, its body moves in sympathy with the motion of the water. To detect sound, a mechanism is required that will cause the cilia bundles above the hair cells in the inner ear of the fish to bend. For this to happen, something in the ear must remain stationary.

On each side of the fish's head there are three dense calcareous masses called otoliths (Figure 8.8). The otoliths are suspended in liquid alongside sensory tissue bearing the cilia bundles of the hair cells. So, although the soft parts of the fish, and much of the hearing mechanism, move with the water when a sound

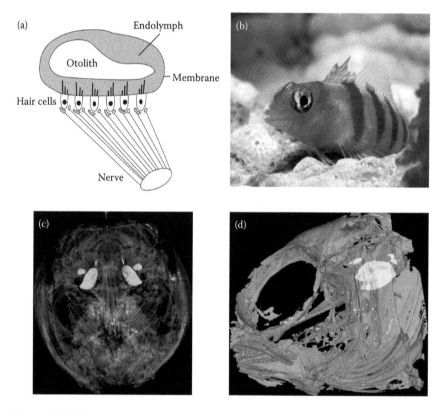

Figure 8.8 (a) A schematic depicting the fish's hearing and balance apparatus in which the calcareous otolith is suspended above the hair cells. Deflection of the cilia above the hair cells when a sound wave passes results in a receptor potential in the hair cells. (Drawing by Vivian L. Ward.) (b) A triplefin photographed at the Poor Knights Islands that is approximately 5 cm long. (c) Frontal view and (d) side view of the head of another triplefin imaged using a micro-CT. Left and right sets of otoliths are visible within the fish's head as the mock color-enhanced green objects. (Micro-CT images courtesy Auckland Bioengineering Institute.)

wave passes, the dense otoliths remain nearly stationary. The displacement of the adjacent hair cells relative to the semi-stationary otoliths bends the cilia bundles along one sensitive direction, generating a signal. At right angles to this direction, there is no response.*

The frequency range for otolithic hearing is in the range of tens to hundreds of hertz and at very small amplitudes [22]. The tiny movements of otolithic hearing can be calculated from behavioral thresholds that show fishes can detect an acoustic pressure of 0.01 Pa at 500 Hz; an amplitude of 2×10^{-12} m. Given that otolithic movement is less than half that of the particle's motion, the stimulus to the receptors must be less than 10^{-12} m at threshold, or about 1/100th the diameter of a hydrogen atom [1]. Ambient noise in the sea increases toward lower frequencies, and turbulence along the edges of ocean currents and seismic motion of the ocean floor could be a source of the high level of ambient infrasound (infrasound is sound at very low frequencies, typically less than 20 Hz). Perhaps the directional pattern of infrasound in the oceans may be an additional cue for navigation.

The directionality of response of individual hair cells and their orientation provide a basis for directional hearing. Two groups of hair cells lying in the same plane and oriented 90° to each other can determine the axis for the direction of a sound within that plane. Adding a third group enables three-dimensional sound direction sensing.

This mechanism provides information to the fish on the axis of the particle motion but does not determine whether the wave is coming from the front or back, for instance. This we call the 180-degree ambiguity. The extra sensing to determine direction of sound, resolving the 180-degree ambiguity, might come from the use of the swim bladder as a sound pressure sensor. When there is some functional connection between the gas-filled cavity of the swim bladder and the inner ear the swim bladder can serve as a means for sound amplification, like a hearing aid, improving hearing sensitivity, and extending the upper frequency range of hearing (up to 2–5 kHz). The sound pressure stimulus derived from the swim bladder on its own cannot provide information on the direction of the source of a sound. However, when combined with information on particle movement, from the otoliths, the phase reference of the pressure could in theory be used to resolve the 180-degree ambiguity [22].

In summary, there are some innovations in hearing that we can borrow from marine mammals and fish. We could, for instance, tune into high-frequency sounds like those of the toothed whales. To make this work we would need receivers that are sensitive in the tens of kilohertz and a way to process the information. This has already been proven to work! Researchers at the National University of Singapore

---

* More precisely, the directional response of the hair cells follows a cosine function—maximal when the motion is aligned with the axis of sensitivity and zero when it is at right angles to the axis.

have demonstrated a wearable set of high-frequency directional receivers that can collect ultrasound in real time, compress the sound from high (20–200 kHz) to lower audible frequencies (1.7–17.7 kHz) and play it back to the diver through headphones. This provided interaural time and intensity differences that were effective in introducing a sense of directional hearing for a person under water [23].

However, for audible mid- to low frequencies, directionality using conventional technology requires hydrophones set meters apart. A towed-array of sufficient length to gain sound directionality, especially for low frequencies, is hardly a realistic option for a diver. To plug this gap we could look to the fish: developing an artificial sensor that is inherently directional like a fish's ear.

And then through the combined working of otolith-like vector sensing and direct pressure sensing from a gas-filled device, inspired by the swim bladder we could potentially resolve the 180-degree ambiguity.

But perhaps the most important advance of all would be to remove the noise of the regulator so we could hear the sounds of the reef. We can do this now, using rebreather technology. Combined with enhanced hearing and directional sensing for navigation we could improve the overall experience. A dive would be like a walk through a forest, not only seeing the natural beauty but also hearing it as well: with fish sounds and dolphin calls in the place of bird song.

References

1. Rogers, P.H. and Cox, M. Underwater sound as a biological stimulus, in *Sensory Biology of Aquatic Animals*, J. Atema, R.R. Fay, A.N. Popper, and W.N. Tavolga Editors. 1988, New York, NY: Springer-Verlag. pp. 131–149.
2. Weirathmueller, M.J., Wilcock, W.S.D., and Soule, D.C. Source levels of fin whale 20 Hz pulses measured in the Northeast Pacific Ocean. *Journal of the Acoustical Society of America*, 2013. 133(2): 741–749.
3. Payne, R. and Webb, D. Orientation by means of long range acoustic signaling in baleen whales. *Annals of the New York Academy of Sciences*, 1971. 188(1): 110–141.
4. Hildebrand, J. Anthropogenic and natural sources of ambient noise in the ocean. *Marine Ecology Progress Series*, 2009. 395: 5–20.
5. Croll, D.A., Clark, C.W., Acevedo, A., Tershy, B., Flores, S., Gedamke, J., and Urban, J. Only male fin whales sing loud songs. *Nature*, 2002. 417: 809.
6. Hildebrand, J.A. Anthropogenic and natural sources of ambient noise in the ocean. *Marine Ecology Progress Series*, 2009. 395: 5–20.
7. Radford, C., Jeffs, A., Tindle, C., and Montgomery, J.C. Resonating sea urchin skeletons create coastal choruses. *Marine Ecology Progress Series*, 2008. 362: 37–43.
8. Radford, C.A., Ghazali, S., Jeffs, A.G., and Montgomery, J.C. Vocalisations of the bigeye, *Pempheris adspersa*: Characteristics, source level, and active space. *Journal of Experimental Biology*, 2015. 218: 940–948.
9. Montgomery, J.C., Jeffs, A., Simpson, S.D., Meekan, M., and Tindle, C. Sound as an orientation cue for the pelagic larvae of reef fishes and decapod crustaceans. *Advances in Marine Biology*, 2006. 51: 143–196.

10. Parvin, S.J. and Nedwell, J.R. Underwater sound perception and the development of an underwater noise weighting scale. *Underwater Technology: The International Journal of the Society for Underwater*, 1995. 21(1): 12–19.

11. Enger, P.S. Hearing in herring. *Comparative Biochemistry and Physiology*, 1967. 22(2): 527–538.

12. Johnson, S.C. Sound detection thresholds in marine mammals, in *Marine Bio-Acoustic*, W. Talvoga, Editor. 1967, New York, NY: Pergamon Press. pp. 247–260.

13. Knudsen, E.I. and Konishi, M. Mechanisms of sound localization in the barn owl (*Tyto alba*). *Journal of Comparative Physiology*, 1979. 133(1): 13–21.

14. Jeffress, L.A. A place theory of sound localization. *Journal of Comparative and Physiological Psychology*, 1948. 41(1): 35–39.

15. Li, G., Tousi, Y.M., Hassibi, A., and Afshari, E. Delay-line-based analog-to-digital converters. *Circuits and Systems II: Express Briefs, IEEE Transactions on*, 2009. 56(6): 464–468.

16. Hartmann, W.M. How we localize sound. *Physics Today*, 1999. 52(11): 24–29 (http://dx.doi.org/10.1063/1.882727).

17. Shupak, A., Sharoni, Z., Yanir, Y., Keynan, Y., Alfie, Y., and Halpern, P. Underwater hearing and sound localization with and without an air interface. *Otology & Neurotology*, 2005. 26(1): 127–130.

18. Hemilä, S., Nummela, S., and Reuter, T. Anatomy and physics of the exceptional sensitivity of dolphin hearing (Odontoceti: Cetacea). *Journal of Comparative Physiology A*, 2010. 196(3): 165–179.

19. Branstetter, B.K. and Mercado, E.I. Sound localization by cetaceans. *International Journal of Comparative Psychology*, 2006. 19(1): 26–61.

20. Johnson, M., Madsen, P.T., Zimmer, W.M.X., de Soto, N.A., and Tyack, P.L. Beaked whales echolocate on prey. *Proceedings of the Royal Society of London B (Suppl.)*, 2004. 271: S383–S386.

21. Leighton, T.G., Chua, G.H., and White, P.R. Do dolphins benefit from nonlinear mathematics when processing their sonar returns? *Proceedings of the Royal Society A*, 2012. doi: 10.1098/rspa.2012.0247.

22. Popper, A.N. and Fay, R.R. The auditory periphery in fishes, in *Comparative Hearing: Fish and Amphibians*, R.R. Fay and A.N. Popper, Editors. 1999, New York, NY: Springer-Verlag. pp. 43–100.

23. Teong-Beng, K., Soo Pieng, T., Soon Keat, Y., Tay, H., Chitre, M., and Potter, J.R. Enabling humans to hear the direction of sounds underwater—Experiments and preliminary results, in *OCEANS 2008*. 2008: 1–9. doi.: 10.1109/OCEANS.2008.5152074.

Chapter 9 Underwater sensing for navigation and survival

Where is the boat? This question is on many an underwater explorer's mind at dive's end. If underwater visibility matched that of air, navigation over several hundred meters would not be an issue; but even in clear tropical water a diver can see barely 100 m, and much less than this in temperate waters made murky by plankton. For the sport diver, the underwater compass is the primary tool for keeping track of direction. To succeed, compass navigation must be supplemented by visual recognition of underwater features (caves, walls, etc.) and "dead reckoning" techniques such as counting one's fin kicks along a specific compass bearing. The sight of the boat's anchor chain at the end of a dive is a welcome reward for good navigation. With our eyes and with a compass on the wrist we can at least avoid becoming dangerously lost.

An obvious question from yachtsmen and hikers would be: why not use a global positioning system (GPS)? The simple answer is that radio waves at the frequencies used for sensing the position of a satellite are strongly attenuated by water. So in the absence of a GPS, what other options are available to us? How do animals navigate in this environment? Lobsters can find home across kilometers of seabed, sea turtles can swim hundreds of kilometers to a beach, and large fish such as the whale shark and great white shark can migrate across the open ocean. Are their senses sharper than ours? Does the world look different? Do some animals have an additional sense?

The answer to all of the above is yes! Sound is an ideal cue for navigational sensing, as was discussed in the last chapter. Other senses include vision, taste, and smell and the ability to detect electric and magnetic fields.

Vision

Much of our navigation depends on recognizing a familiar underwater landscape, which depends on good illumination. As we dive deeper the light levels go down, but this loss is not evenly spread across the spectrum. Colors at the long wavelength (red) end of the visual spectrum are lost first, which happens in relatively

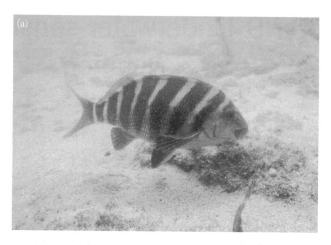

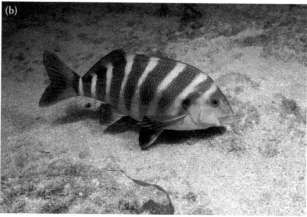

Figure 9.1 A red moki (*Cheilodactylus spectabilis*) at 5 m depth, photographed (a) in natural light and (b) with an underwater flash at the Goat Island Marine Reserve, Leigh. (Photos by Iain A. Anderson.)

shallow water (Figure 9.1). If you cut yourself at 10 m depth, your blood will look green in the ambient light; illumination by a torch will confirm that you are indeed bleeding red blood and that you should leave the water before you attract unwanted attention from something big.

The shallow, sunlit upper part of the water column that we visit is also the region penetrated by sunlight where most of the ocean's food production occurs. This is the photic zone. The end point of the photic zone is usually defined as the depth at which attenuation reduces photon flux density to only 1% of the surface value. Photic zone depths can vary between 10 and several hundred meters [1], subject to daily or even hourly change in the density, depth, and composition of plankton and suspended organic materials. Despite this variation in light attenuation, some large creatures can use light levels for vertical navigation. There is good evidence for this from one of the rarest sharks: the megamouth (*Megachasma pelagios*).

The megamouth is a deepwater shark, described as large (~5 m long) and flabby with a very big mouth and rubbery lips that it uses for capturing plankton. The very first megamouth shark to have drawn scientific attention was caught in Hawaii in 1976; there have been only 50 or so specimens caught or seen since then, so we know little about the shark. An analysis of the anatomy of the megamouth suggests that it has a mode of feeding that involves a combination of actively sucking the prey into its cavernous mouth and then assisting this with ram feeding: driving more water into its mouth by swimming forward [2]. The sixth known specimen of a megamouth captured and released in 1990 off the Californian coast provided insight into this shark's ability to follow light levels [2]. Using acoustic transmitters attached to the shark, researchers followed its movements for just over 2 days. On release it moved in a relatively straight path at a speed of just over 0.3 m/s, although its speed relative to the water was probably higher since it was swimming against a current. During this period, the shark spent the day from sunrise to sunset at about 140 m, and the night from sunset to sunrise at about 20 m. These daytime/nighttime depths were associated with the same specific intensity of light, suggesting that the shark was using light levels for vertical navigation.

Perhaps it was following the zooplankton. At night, zooplankton rise from depths of more than 200 m (in the open ocean), and feed on phytoplankton [3] (single-celled dinoflagellates, diatoms, and cyanobacteria) that have spent the daylight hours near the surface producing food using photosynthesis. Zooplankton prefer low light levels associated with depth, avoiding predators, but will come up to the surface if conditions are right, and a dark night is favorable for this. One author (IAA) has observed zooplankton-rich water suddenly becoming sparse on the rising of the moon. There might also be a nutritional advantage for the zooplankton to leave the phytoplankton alone during the day, as this would allow food reserves to build up at the surface [4]. A planktivore, like a megamouth, would benefit from navigating on absolute light levels to keep in step with its food source. This would seem to be what a megamouth is doing.

Across the animal kingdom the ability to sense light is widespread. It is clear that the creatures of the zooplankton can differentiate between day and night and some have quite complex light-sensitive organs. In the much larger scyphozoan and cubozoan jellyfish (refer to Chapter 4), these are found in control centers (rhopalia) on the rim of the bell. Rhopalia also have gravity-sensing organs and neural pacemaker circuitry, which initiate contraction of the bell. The most complex jellyfish eye organs belong to the box jellyfish: the Cubomedusans (Figure 9.2). Each has 24 eyes of 4 different types: 2, like ours, contain the equivalent of a light-sensing

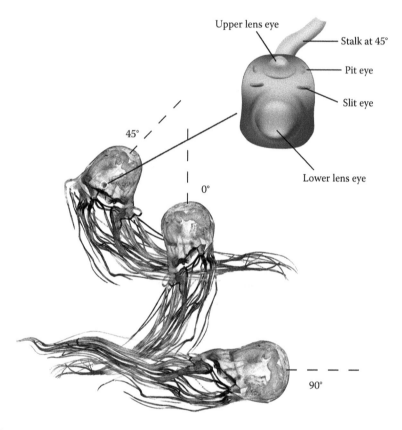

Figure 9.2 A box jellyfish in three orientations. Box jellyfish have four rhopalia each with six eyes and a statolith at the base. The flexible stalk allows the rhopalium to maintain its vertical orientation, despite the position of the jellyfish, so that the upper eye lens is always looking up. (After Coates, M.M., *Integrative and Comparative Biology*, 43(4), 542–548, 2003 [7].) (Drawing by Mark T. Ryan.)

retina, and a cornea, pupil, and lens to direct the image onto the retina [5]. The eye types serve different functions that might require less neural processing than if all the visual information had to travel through the same eye [6]. One of the two camera-like eyes, the upper lens eye, might play a key role in navigation. As its name suggests, this eye is always looking upward; this is ensured by a simple ballast mechanism: each rhopalium carries a cell (statocyst) with a ballast weight so that it is orientated the same way despite the swimming direction of the animal. Although the lens could potentially bring an image to focus, the retina is located too close to the lens for this to happen.

The result is that the retina receives an image that is blurred but still sufficient for navigation. Perhaps the most agile of the box jellies is the species (*Tripedalia cystophora*). The swimming response of this box jellyfish to changes in lighting direction has been studied using tethered animals in an aquarium [8]. Turning the light source off on one of the four sides produced swimming responses causing the jellyfish to use its velarium, a ring of tissue that focuses the jet, to swim away from the dark direction and toward the light [9]. This box jellyfish inhabits mangrove swamps. Through this light sensitivity it is able to maintain position between, or near to, mangroves [6] enabling the jellyfish to find and feed on small crustacea that congregate in shafts of light between the trees and to avoid contact with mangrove roots and wharf pilings that cast shadows.

Looking directly up through shallow, relatively still and clear water a jellyfish eye will receive a 180° view of the scene above the water. But due to the way in which light rays bend, or refract, at the air/water interface, this panoramic view is contracted into an area known as Snell's window (Figure 9.3). Outside the zone of Snell's window, beyond an angle of about 48° from the vertical, the air/water interface acts like a mirror and typically appears dark. Lying on your back in a mangrove estuary you will see within Snell's window nearby trees as dark shapes toward the edge of the window; useful cues for maintaining position by the jellyfish.

These examples show how we can control behavior economically using dedicated eye structures, how to navigate by simply looking up (box jellyfish), and how a blurred image can be used for navigation and sensing (box jellyfish, scallop).

To see details in objects requires the sharp focusing of an image onto the photosensitive neurons of a retina. As light enters an animal's eye it is refracted by the cornea, the "main image-forming component" [10], with additional focusing by the lens. Our eye is configured to work in the air and our cornea acts as a lens. But underwater, the cornea is ineffective because the index of refraction of the cornea is approximately the same as water. To focus underwater we therefore require an air interface between water and eye, normally provided by goggles or facemask.

Fish have eyes similar to ours but they can focus underwater. With the cornea not capable of effectively focusing light the lens takes over the primary role of focusing. The lens of the fish eye is spherical, providing as short a focal length as possible (Figure 9.4). If the lens were composed of the same material throughout it would suffer severe spherical aberration: light rays arriving at the edges of the lens would be overfocused and light near the axis would be underfocused (Figure 9.5). Therefore, to correct for this and instead of adding another optical element in the field, fish have a solution: a lens with a gradient of refractive index from center to the edge; high at the center and reducing to the edge. A light ray at the edge will therefore be bent less and all parallel rays can come to a single focus (Figure 9.5). Such a lens with its spherical symmetry has a great advantage in that there is no single axis for light to pass through (as in the human eye) and the image is

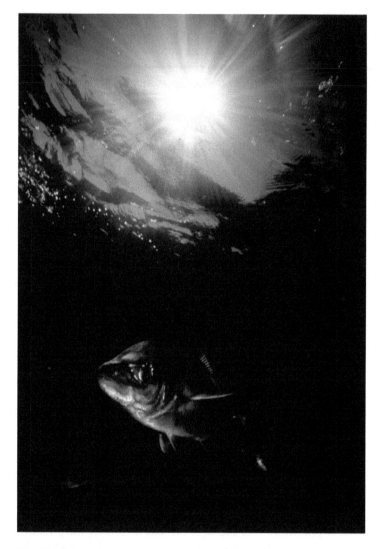

Figure 9.3 This trevally (*Caranx georgianus*) in the Poor Knights Islands is lit up from below by the photographer's flash. In the background, we see sunlight through Snell's window. (Photo by Iain A. Anderson.)

well resolved over a wide field [10]. Cetaceans (whales) and pinnipeds (seals) also have spherical or near spherical lenses, and in cetaceans at least the lenses are also nonhomogeneous, like fish eyes [11].

Both pinnipeds and cetaceans spend time in dark and deep water. To compensate for this, their eyes have a reflective structure (*tapetum lucidum*) behind the retina

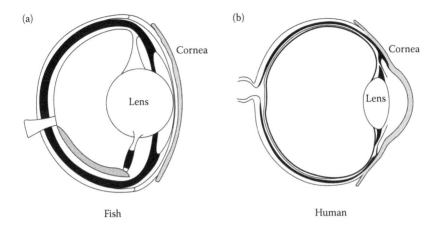

Figure 9.4 Schematic of a fish eye with its spherical lens (a) and a human eye (b). (Drawing by Vivian L. Ward.)

that reflects light back across the retina [11] and this increases the light that is available to photoreceptors. It works as a quarter wavelength or Bragg mirror; described below. Thus, light passes in both directions. Pinnipeds and cetaceans share such structures with many nocturnal animals that include cats, dogs, raccoons, and fish. It was the reflections from a cat's eye in the headlamp of Percy Shaw's car that gave him the inspiration for the cat's eye reflective road marker [12].

In some animals, sight is based on reflective rather than refractive optics. Our largest optical telescopes use an objective mirror that brings light to a focus enabling us to see the faintest galaxies and other deep sky objects. Mirror lensing is already in use in the sea [13]: the most interesting part of the scallop, which you are not served in the restaurant, is the 60–100 mirror optic eyes that, in the live animal, stare back at you from between the open shells (Figure 9.6). As recently as the mid-1960s, it was assumed that their eyes used refractive elements. This was wrong as highlighted by Land's description of what he saw when he looked into a scallop eye: "an inverted image of the room, including a distorted image of myself looking through the microscope" [10, p. 442]. This could only have been formed by the silvery mirror lining the back of the eye. Unlike our telescope mirrors that have a reflective coating of aluminum or silver, the scallop mirror is a Bragg mirror, produced by layering materials with different refractive index one atop the other (Figure 9.7). Light within a narrow band around a specific wavelength will be very effectively reflected if the optical path for each layer is equal to a quarter wavelength of the light. In the scallop's eyes, the two materials are crystals of guanine (refractive index 1.83) and cytoplasm (refractive index 1.33) with 5 pairs of layers/μm, each layer about 0.1 μm thick, and reflecting green light (500–550 nm) [10]. The lens is

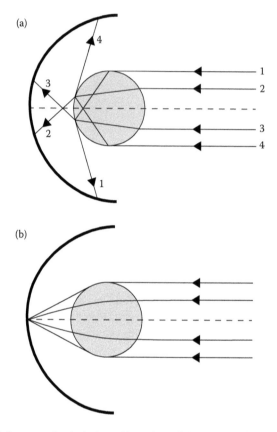

Figure 9.5 (a) Severe spherical aberration where light rays arriving at the edges of the lens are overfocused and light rays near the axis are underfocused. (b) A solution to the fish eye problem—a lens that through a gradient of refractive index, using added proteins, is able to bring underwater light to a focus. (After Land, M.F. *Contemporary Physics*, 29(5), 435–455, 1988 [10].) (Redrawn by Vivian L. Ward.)

also in contact with the retina; there is no space between the two so light that is focused at the top of the retina passes through the retina twice. This will be bad for image contrast. But the scallop needs only to see changes in light intensity, so the top of the retina where the image is focused responds to light going off (predator approaching). The scallop's response includes shutting its shell and escape-jetting by rapidly opening and closing the shell.

The eyes of shrimp, crayfish, and lobsters (decapod crustaceans) (Figure 9.8) demonstrate how light can be directed toward a retina-like sensor array using flat mirrors [10]. They have a type of compound eye that consists of arrays of separate

(a)

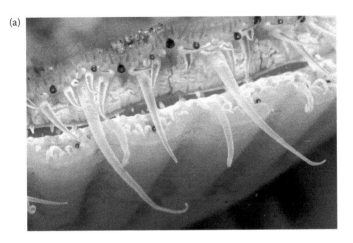

(b)

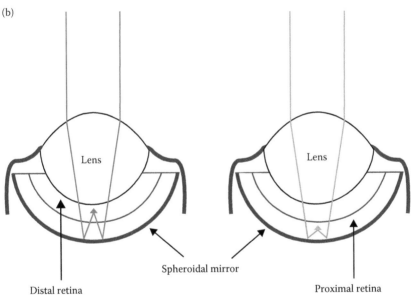

Figure 9.6 (a) A close-up photo of a scallop showing its eyes. (Photos by Iain A. Anderson.) (b) Schematic of the optical system for the scallop eye. There are two retinas each with a different visual pigment. The distal retina, closest to the lens might be sensitive to longer wavelengths of light than the proximal retina. This might be a mechanism to compensate for chromatic aberration when a lens is unable to bring all wavelengths of light to the same focus. (From Speiser, D.I., Loew, E.R., and Johnsen, S. *Journal of Experimental Biology*, 214(3), 422–431, 2011 [14].) (Drawing by Iain A. Anderson.)

(a) (b)

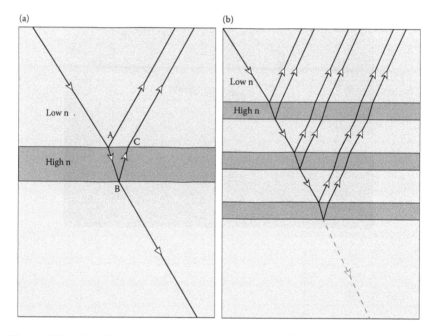

Figure 9.7 (a) A light beam traveling from low to high refractive index material is partially reflected and partially transmitted at A. At the interface, the reflected ray undergoes a 180° phase shift. The transmitted ray after passing through a quarter wavelength thickness is partially reflected at B. The reflected ray joins the surface ray and is in phase with it. (b) Multiple layers of high and low index material can be stacked to return much of the incident beam. (Drawings by Iain A. Anderson.)

lensing elements that collectively provide an ultrawide field of view. Compound eye design is a rich area for exploration; for more complete accounts the reader is referred to the reviews by Nilsson [15] and Land [10].

The optical elements of decapod crustacean compound eyes are known as ommatidia. A close-up photograph of a decapod's eye reveals a multifaceted square grid pattern. Each optical element or ommatidium resembles four flat-faced truncated pyramids with mirrored surfaces. A ray of light that passes into an ommatidium is reflected by up to two of its internal mirrored surfaces that then direct it toward a rhabdom, a rod-like organ containing photoreceptor cells. Rhabdoms are arrayed behind the cornea on a retina-like structure within the eye. Any two mirrored surfaces that are at right angles to each other will return a light ray in a plane that is parallel to the plane of the incident ray (Figure 9.9).

Light rays emanating from a point source and arriving at other ommatidia can be brought together, or superposed, onto the same rhabdom. This arrangement of mirrors for focusing light has provided inspiration for reflecting optical devices:

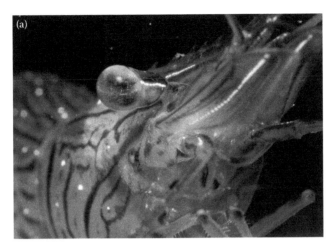

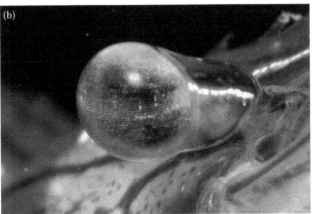

Figure 9.8 (a) The head of a 3 cm long shrimp (*Palaemon affinis*) photographed under a wharf. (b) A close-up of its ultrawide angle reflecting a superposition compound eye. Note the rectangular grid pattern of the ommatidia. (Photos by Iain A. Anderson.)

x-ray telescopes for deep-space research also employ reflecting superposition optics. In these telescopes, high-energy x-rays are focused using nested circular bands of mirrors. X-rays reflect from the mirrors at very small grazing angles. Each mirror set focuses its annulus of x-rays to a common detector. Unlike the decapod eye these designs have very limited fields of view, order of 1° of arc. Over 30 years ago a telescope design based on the decapod rectangular multi-mirror cell was described that could combine the ability to capture high-energy x-rays at low grazing angles over a very wide field of view [16]. "Lobster optics" could

143

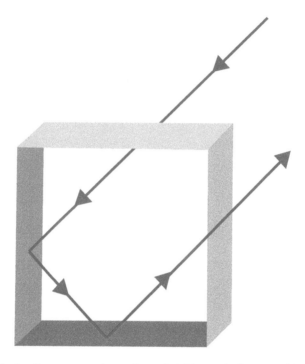

Figure 9.9 In the figure, we portray a box mimicking a single ommatidium with internal reflecting surfaces arranged at right angles (90°) to each other. A light ray entering from the back is double reflected so that it emerges from the front in a plane that is parallel to the incident plane.

enable wide-field surveys of the x-ray sky from small satellites [17], and they could be applied to imaging in the visible spectrum too, providing extremely wide fields of view in a compact assembly (Figure 9.10) [18].

The compound eye of the mantis shrimp provides an interesting contrast to the decapod eye. Mantis shrimps (Figure 9.11) are known for their ability to rapidly impale or crush prey at close range using praying mantis-like forelimbs. To accurately land blows they must have the ability to find the range to the target using eyes that stand prominently on stalks and that are separately steerable.

We need both of our eyes to judge range but mantis shrimps might be able to measure range with only one eye [19]. To understand how they do this we consider the functional structure of the mantis shrimp eye.

Light that enters the eye passes through the cornea into each ommatidium within which there is a lens-like structure, the crystalline cone, which directs light by refraction (rather than reflection) onto the rhabdom with its photosensitive cells.

144

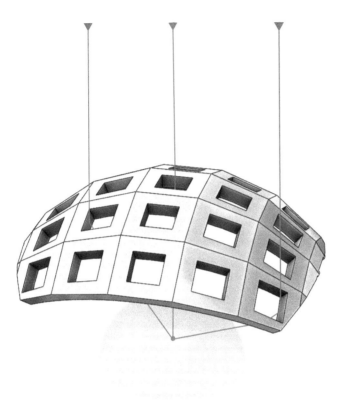

Figure 9.10 A hypothetical multi-mirror wide field of view compound lensing system. Here, we depict three parallel rays that come to focus on a light-sensing element on the hemisphere. The bottom right-hand side ray is doubly reflected in the manner indicated in Figure 9.9. (After Huang, C.-C. et al. *Small*, 10(15), 3050–3057, 2014 [18].)

Each rhabdom receives light from its own section of cornea so that an ommatidium operates as an optically isolated unit [15]. This is the basic plan for the compound apposition eye, unlike the compound superposition eye of the shrimp and lobster described above that can channel light from several ommatidia to a rhabdom. Superposition optics are superior for gathering light. But the apposition eye offers some advantages when it comes to range-finding and other specializations that have been exploited by the mantis shrimp.

The hexagonal ommatidia of the mantis shrimp are arranged into two hemispheres separated by mid-band rows with enlarged hexagonal facets [20]. Species of mantis shrimp that inhabit well-lit colorful shallows of tropical surface waters have a prominent mid-band with 6 rows of ommatidia supporting 14 different

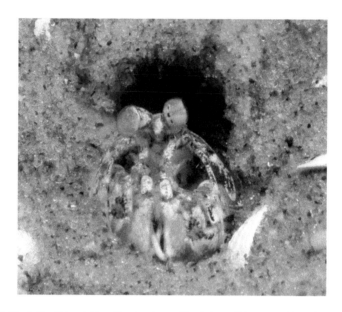

Figure 9.11 A Northland New Zealand mantis shrimp (*Heterosquilla tricarinata*) living in the sand in Whangateau Harbor in its usual pose, looking out of its burrow with its eyes turning independently. The hexagonal ommatidia of the mantis shrimp eye are arranged into two hemispheres separated by mid-band rows with enlarged hexagonal facets. Each provides a light path to a single rhabdom. This arrangement is visible on the shrimp's left-hand side eye. This is not visible on the shrimp's right-hand side eye that has been rotated about 90° to the left eye. The field of view for ommatidia on opposing sides of the mid-band overlap and this provides a means for distance to target ranging within the same eye. Good ranging is required for accurate aim of their sharp spine covered forelimbs. Opening the limbs exposes the sharp spines. The animal makes its "strike" by spearing its prey with its open limbs. Prey can be impaled on their spines in less than 100th of a second. (Photo by Iain A. Anderson.)

photoreceptor cell types. Central bands of ommatidia have their longitudinal axes skewed so that instead of tilting around to follow the curvature of the eyeball they maintain optical alignment that results in substantial visual overlap between both hemispheres. The result is that 70% of the eye views a narrow strip in space.

The apposition compound eye has also inspired the development of wrap around sensor arrays that can provide a panoramic field of view for motion detection [21].

Range-finding is made possible by image overlap: when ommatidia on both sides of the mid-band of the same eye receive light from the same point. The mid-band rows equip them with 12-channel color vision enabling them to see evenly through the spectrum from 300 nm wavelength (ultraviolet) to 720 nm wavelength (red) [22] and there are photoreceptors within the mid-bands that provide sensitivity to polarized light.* To gather information around them their eyes are in almost continuous and independent motion, rapidly scanning the environment [22]. Mantis shrimps are clearly sensitive to color, which is useful for image recognition in shallow water so that polarized light might enhance their ability to see detail in objects [23,24]. Light reflecting off of dielectric (nonconducting) surfaces will be polarized. Perhaps this helps the shrimp to identify friends or foes.

Cephalopods (octopus, squid, cuttlefish) also discriminate polarized light; through the orthogonal arrangement of their retinal photoreceptors. Cuttlefish and octopus can see polarized light, react to it and even reflect it from their bodies, using it as a behavioral cue [25].

Much of the ambient light beneath the surface of the sea is polarized and if it can be detected it could be used as a navigation tool [26]. Sunlight striking the surface is polarized when refracted into the water and polarized light from the sky (celestial) can also be detected within Snell's window. But for celestial and solar light to provide a means for navigation, waters would ideally be shallow, clear and calm, quite a rare combination of conditions. Whether or not cephalopods use it directly for navigation is under debate. But their sensitivity to polarized light might improve their ability to see under conditions of low visibility associated with turbid and murky water [27].

Many reef dwellers and humans rely on vision for navigating over short distances, order of a hundred meters, but over longer distances vision as a tool for navigation is limited, unless we look down to retrace our path over familiar scenery. This option is not available to creatures living in the open ocean where the average depth exceeds a kilometer. In the previous chapter we described how sound can be used for navigating on the kilometer scale. There is also scent (olfaction) for long-distance navigation.

Scent

Spear fishermen occasionally encounter sharks that are drawn to the blood of a speared fish. Like other fish, sharks have a very well-developed olfactory sense. And scents can be distributed rapidly over long distances, carried along by tides and currents.

The ability to track chemicals in water or air can find use in a number of areas including environmental management (tracking to the source of a pollutant), gas pipeline leaks, health monitoring of underwater equipment, and of course

_____

* Light (and other electromagnetic radiation) is characterized by two orthogonal fields magnetic (M) and electric (E). Nonpolarized light is characterized by a random e-vector orientation. Light is polarized when its e-vector vibrates predominately in one plane or rotates in one direction. Polarization can be produced by reflection from a dielectric surface.

navigation. Swimming robots equipped with chemical sensors can be used in toxic or dangerous environments that are unsafe for humans [28]. But how should a robot be programed to correctly interpret the sampled data in a gas or liquid chemical plume that is subject to slow diffusion or perhaps in turbulent flow composed of intermittent and broken eddies?

There are many examples ranging from microscopic bacteria (refer to Chapter 2) to much larger organisms that include crustaceans [29]. For organisms that move at very low Reynolds numbers (Re) (refer to Chapter 2), much less than one, such as bacteria, diffusion is the principal mechanism for the transfer of chemical signals: such organisms employ strategies such as helical klinotaxis for tracking the location of nutrients (see Chapter 2). As fluid velocity and length scale increase (higher Re) the fluid's bulk motion becomes increasingly important as a means for transporting chemical signals. And laminar flow, where there is little or no mixing, gives way to turbulent flow; rough surfaces on the seabed combined with very much higher Re flow (Re $> 10^4$–10^6) favor turbulent conditions, through which larger animals such as crabs must navigate. For them, chemical information is carried in fast moving plumes that are intermittent and that also mix and dilute the chemical. But although they move about at higher Re their antennae with their finely structured setae (refer to Chapter 2) operate at much lower Re so that the speed at which they flick the antennae through the fluid is important for sampling; this is discussed by Koehl [30] (refer to Chapter 2).

They also face the same challenges as any robotic sniffing device would. A chemical plume, downstream from a food source or a potential mate, can be very difficult to read if the flow is turbulent and irregular; with big changes in concentration density over short distances and times. Rather than relying on the intensity of an odor, sharks use an odor pulse's arrival time and position relative to nearest nostril to provide a cue for navigating toward the odor source [31]. Crustaceans instead use spatial sampling techniques: differences in response from chemical sensors distributed across their bodies can be used to determine their position relative to the chemical plume and they move sideways and forward, positioning themselves in the flow [29]. Perhaps they are forming a mental map of the plume. Experiments have been conducted with crabs in controlled flow downstream of the artificial scent of a clam. The results suggest that flow is good for giving a clue to the direction of a chemical source. But if the flow is too fast then the scent plumes might be too narrow and missed altogether. If too slow then success is poor [32]. Being in a strong flow might also have some survival advantages: a strong flow will be less likely to betray one's position to an adversary or predator.

How salmon navigate at sea is not known, but once back at the coast, they recognize the distinctive scent signature of their home river, where they were spawned using a mind map. As they migrate up the river, each confluence, or side stream entering the river, provides a choice. That choice is also made on the basis of scent [33]. We assume that if the scent above the confluence does not match the memory they have of the scents experienced on their downriver migration as juveniles, then they cease their upstream movement and drop back below the confluence and make that choice again. Therefore, it is believed that their homing to the stream in which they were spawned is a result of replaying the scent memory trace they set down during their initial downstream migration.

Electrical and magnetic fields

The ability to sense electric field sets sharks, and their cousins, the rays and chimaeras, apart from most other fish. Their electrosensory system not only provides the ability to see prey in the dark or buried in the sand but potentially enables global positioning. Their electrical sense organs (ampullae of Lorenzini) located within pores on the head can detect faint electrical signals with a threshold of 5 nV/cm (Figure 9.12). This is equivalent to the voltage gradient set up by a 1.5 V dry cell battery with its ends 3000 km, apart! The shark and its relatives are able to detect these faint field signals above the noise of their own similar electrical fields up to about 1 m away. This distance may not sound very far, especially given the sensitivity of the system, but the source fields are small, and short circuit in the surrounding seawater. In addition, detection distances of less than a meter are still very useful for hunting in the dark, or discovery of prey buried beneath a thin layer of sand. This is aided by an active noise canceling system in the brain in a structure quite similar to our own cerebellum (refer to Chapter 7). This strategy for noise cancelation is interesting from a biomimetic point of view in that it employs signal/noise improvement strategies that anticipate by 400 million years or so those that are currently used in electrical engineering. These include common-mode suppression and active cancelation such as used in noise-canceling headphones.

Each ampulla is connected to the outside by a tube that penetrates the skin (Figure 9.12). Beneath the skin, the canal is surrounded by cells that are tightly connected to each other giving an impermeable layer. At the end of the canal in the ampulla are the receptor cells, probably modified from the mechanosensory hair cells found in the lateral line and the hearing organs (refer to Chapter 8). Only a small part of the receptor cell is exposed to the canal. The whole system is filled with an electrically conducting gel and surrounded by an electrically insulating layer. Externally, a small prey item acts as an electric dipole. When it is close to the fish the ampullae detect the voltage drop through the thickness of the skin. How they do this is complex, but it involves transport of calcium ions (Ca^{2+}) into the sensory cell, promoting release of a neurotransmitter, and depolarization of the nerve fiber-carrying impulses toward the central nervous system (e.g., afferent

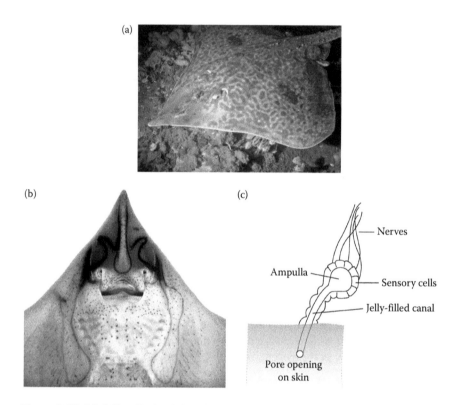

Figure 9.12 (a) A New Zealand thornback ray photographed near Aramoana. (Photo by Kim Westerskov.) (b) The underside head region of a thornback ray. The lateral lines have been filled with blue ink (injection site on the left side of the photo). The black dots are the natural pigmentation around the openings of the ampullae of Lorenzini, each a jelly-filled canal. Some of the cells lining this canal are electro-receptive with the ability to detect potential differences between the pore and the base. (c) A schematic of an ampulla of Lorenzini. (Drawing by Vivian L. Ward.)

fiber), resulting in a nervous impulse. Mimicking the sensitivity of this system is perhaps beyond the capability of our current technologies.

Even if we cannot easily mimic the electrosense, it might be possible to use it for driving sharks away: for example, an electrical shark repellent. Devices for doing this include the Shark Shield, an electronic power pack strapped to the leg with a 2 meter long cable behind that sends out a pulsed electric field. According to the patent [34], the electrical signal serves to "over-stimulate the nervous system of a shark." There is some evidence that they do influence the shark's behavior, although it is debated as to how effective they might be in protecting a diver from attack [35].

The shark electrosense has a possible role to play in global positioning for it is sufficiently sensitive to detect weak electrical fields induced by its own movement through the Earth's magnetic field [36]. This is supported by observations of shark navigational ability. Some sharks can navigate over thousands of kilometers. Whale sharks [37,38] traverse oceans; one wearing a satellite tag traveled over 13,000 km from the eastern Pacific to the Indian Ocean. Great white sharks are also masters of ocean navigation, a tagged shark traveled from the South African coast all the way across to Ningaloo Reef, Western Australia, much of this was a near straight-line migration [39]. The idea is simple (Figure 9.13): the shark's body induces an electrical field due to its movement across the field lines of the Earth's magnetic field. The body of the shark is therefore like a length of conductor being forced past the magnetic field lines of a magnet. The electric field that is induced will be detected by the ampullae of Lorenzini.

For this to work well, we must assume that the water in which it swims is also stationary, which is often not the case. Ocean currents also produce electric fields of similar strength as they too are conductors moving in the Earth's magnetic field. Such fields will also be detected by the shark. So it seems that we cannot attribute the shark's GPS entirely to this simple model. At the very least these stimuli to the electrosensory system provide a compass-like sense of direction, but because the Earth's magnetic field varies in direction with latitude (horizontal

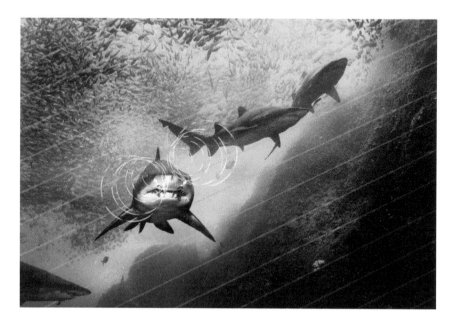

Figure 9.13 As this shark (*Carcharias taurus*) moves through the Earth's magnetic field (parallel green lines), the electric field it induces (white circles) might be sensed by its ampullae of Lorenzini. (Photo and image by Iain A. Anderson.)

near the equator, becoming vertical toward the magnetic poles), this sense may provide some global positioning information.

Whether it is electrosensory or olfactory, a key to navigation over very long distances is the ability to produce a map, to know where you are in relation to where you need to be. Returning to the magnetic field, other animals that lack these electrosensory organs have demonstrated this ability, in particular regarding the Earth's magnetic field.

Sea turtles, for instance, can travel for hundreds of kilometers over apparently featureless ocean to arrive at a specific feeding, nesting, or breeding site, following virtually straight-line paths to their goals. The movements of a female green turtle in the South China Sea were tracked from her nesting beach on an island near Malaysia to her feeding grounds in the North Natuna Archipelago, a distance of 600 km. On the final leg of the journey, she swam 475 km maintaining a near constant speed and direction both day and night [40]. University of North Carolina marine biologists Kenneth and Catherine Lohmann have also demonstrated how loggerhead turtle hatchlings [41] can recognize and orient their swimming to magnetic field direction, while subjected to a controlled magnetic field created using large electromagnetic coils. This device enabled them to simulate the local magnetic field at opposite sides of the Atlantic Ocean. Hatchlings exposed to a field like the one on the eastern Atlantic tried to swim westward and those exposed to a field like the one on the western side swam east. The hatchlings seemed to know which way to swim, relative to the magnetic field, and this could help them remain safely inside the North Atlantic gyre. Despite these navigational abilities, turtles sometimes stray into cold water. Whether this is intentional we do not know, but green turtles land in New Zealand in waters that are too cold considering their normal range. After nursing them back to health their postrelease movements can be tracked.

Lobsters, the first invertebrates to have demonstrated the ability to navigate over unfamiliar terrain back to their "capture" site, can possibly read the magnetic field [42,43]. In a New Zealand study, 32 lobsters were monitored for up to a year using "acoustic tags" fitted to their backs. Most were stay-at-home types, although some were tracked as far as 2–3 km. These wanderers could find their way home, some even to the original den, although to what extent and whether this was entirely due to reading the magnetic field we cannot be sure.

Bacteria have provided a clue for a magnetic sensor mechanism. Some bacteria accumulate hydrogen peroxide as part of their metabolism. If iron is present, it neutralizes the peroxide, which would otherwise be toxic, forming small chains made of spheres of magnetite, which become magnetized as they are formed. The bacteria now tend to swim along the lines of the Earth's magnetic field. The usefulness of magnetite in bacteria, other than as part of a detoxifying mechanism, is open to question, but the realization of the chemistry, and its effect on the behavior and orientation of the bacteria, led biologists to search for a magnetic sensor mechanism. This has been confirmed in most animals examined, although the localization and identification of the magnetoreceptive cells has proved more difficult [44] and likened to searching for a needle in a stack of needles. One way in which the sense may function is for a chain of magnetic spheres, to be tethered at one end by several lines to the cell membrane. As the orientation of the cell changes, due to movements of the animal, the tethers are pulled asymmetrically. The resultant changes in permeability of the membrane could then be transduced into a neuronal signal [45,46].

We should not lose sight of the fact that senses combine to provide homing information. For the lobster, these other senses include smell and sight and it could be that these sensory cues are combined with magnetic sensing to enable navigation. Specific sensory data are never used in isolation but rather combined and processed in some way either locally by ganglia as in the box jellyfish or centrally by a cerebellum-like structure as in the shark. So in our own efforts to navigate from point to point we can take a lesson from this; by combining compass information with visual and other sensory information, and forming a mind map, one day we can confidently find our way back to the boat at the end of every dive.

References

1. Tett, P. The photic zone, in *Light and Life in the Sea*, P.J. Herring, Editor. 1990, Cambridge: Cambridge University Press. 357pp.
2. Nakaya, K., Matsumoto, R., and Suda, K. Feeding strategy of the megamouth shark *Megachasma pelagios* (Lamniformes: Megachasmidae). *Journal of Fish Biology*, 2008. 73(1): 17–34.
3. Waterman, T.H., Nunnemacher R.F., Chase, F.A. Jr., and Clarke G.L. Diurnal vertical migrations of deep-water plankton. *Biological Bulletin*, 1939. 76: 256–279.
4. Harris, J.E. Physical factors involved in the vertical migration of plankton. *Quarterly Journal of Microscopical Science*, 1953. 94(4): 537–550.
5. O'Connor, M., Garm, A., and Nilsson, D.-E. Structure and optics of the eyes of the box jellyfish *Chiropsella bronzie*. *Journal of Comparative Physiology A*, 2009. 195(6): 557–569.
6. Garm, A., Oskarsson, M., and Nilsson, D.-E. Box Jellyfish use terrestrial visual cues for navigation. *Current Biology: CB*, 2011. 21(9): 798–803.
7. Coates, M.M. Visual ecology and functional morphology of Cubozoa (Cnidaria). *Integrative and Comparative Biology*, 2003. 43(4): 542–548.
8. Ronald Petie, A.G. and Nilsson, D.-E. Visual control of steering in the box jellyfish *Tripedalia cystophora*. *Journal of Experimental Biology*, 2011. 214: 2809–2815.
9. Stöckl, A.L., Petie, R., and Nilsson, D.-E. Setting the pace: New insights into central pattern generator interactions in box jellyfish swimming. *PLoS One*, 2011. 6(11): e27201.
10. Land, M.F. The optics of animal eyes. *Contemporary Physics*, 1988. 29(5): 435–455.
11. Mass, A.M. and Supin, A.Y.A. Adaptive features of aquatic mammals' eye. *Anatomical Record: Advances in Integrative Anatomy and Evolutionary Biology*, 2007. 290(6): 701–715.

153

12. Colvile, R. Percy Shaw: Man with his eye on the road. *The Telegraph.* November 30, 2007, Telegraph Media Group Ltd.
13. Land, M.F. Eyes with mirror optics. *Journal of Optics A: Pure and Applied Optics,* 2000. 2(6): R44.
14. Speiser, D.I., Loew, E.R., and Johnsen, S. Spectral sensitivity of the concave mirror eyes of scallops: Potential influences of habitat, self-screening and longitudinal chromatic aberration. *Journal of Experimental Biology,* 2011. 214(3): 422–431.
15. Nilsson, D.-E. Optics and evolution of the compound eye, in *Facets of Vision,* D. Stavenga and R. Hardie, Editors. 1989, Berlin, Heidelberg: Springer. pp. 30–73.
16. Angel, J.R.P. Lobster eyes as X-ray telescopes. *Astrophysical Journal,* 1979. 233(1): 364–373.
17. Pina, L., Burrows, D., Cash, W., Cerna, D., Gorenstein, P., Hudec, R., Inneman, A. et al. X-ray monitoring for astrophysical applications. *Proceedings of SPIE 9207, Advances in X-ray/EUV Optics and Components IX,* September 5, 2014.
18. Huang, C.-C., Wu, X., Liu, H., Aldalali, B., Rogers, J.A., and Jiang, H. Large-field-of-view wide-spectrum artificial reflecting superposition compound eyes. *Small,* 2014. 10(15): 3050–3057.
19. Schiff, H., Abbott, B.C., and Manning, R.B. Possible monocular range-finding mechanisms in stomatopods from different environmental light conditions. *Comparative Biochemistry and Physiology Part A: Physiology,* 1985. 80(3): 271–280.
20. Marshall, J., Cronin, T.W., and Kleinlogel, S. Stomatopod eye structure and function: A review. *Arthropod Structure & Development,* 2007. 36(4): 420–448.
21. Floreano, D., Pericet-Camara, R., Viollet, S., Ruffier, F., Brückner, A., Leitel, R., Buss, W. et al. Miniature curved artificial compound eyes. *Proceedings of the National Academy of Sciences,* 2013. 110(23): 9267–9272.
22. Marshall, N., Land, M., and Cronin, T. Shrimps that pay attention: Saccadic eye movements in stomatopod crustaceans. *Philosophical Transactions of the Royal Society B.* 369: 20130042.
23. Cronin, T.W. and Marshall, J. Patterns and properties of polarized light in air and water. *Philosophical Transactions of the Royal Society B: Biological Sciences,* 2011. 366(1565): 619–626.
24. Cronin, T.W., Shashar, N., Caldwell, R.L., Marshall, J., Cheroske, A.G., and Chiou, T-H. Polarization vision and its role in biological signaling. *Integrative and Comparative Biology,* 2003. 43(4): 549–558.
25. Shashar, N., Rutledge, P.S., and Cronin, T.W. Polarization vision in cuttlefish—A concealed communication channel? *Journal of Experimental Biology,* 1996. 199: 2077–2084.
26. Lerner, A., Sabbah, S., Erlick, C., and Shashar, N. Navigation by light polarization in clear and turbid waters. *Philosophical Transactions of the Royal Society B: Biological Sciences,* 2011. 366(1565): 671–679.
27. Cartron, L., Josef, N., Lerner, A., McCusker, S.D., Darmaillacq, A-S., Dickel, L., and Shashar, N. Polarization vision can improve object detection in turbid waters by cuttlefish. *Journal of Experimental Marine Biology and Ecology,* 2013. 447: 80–85.
28. Ishida, H., Wada, Y., and Matsukura, H. Chemical sensing in robotic applications: A review. *IEEE Sensors Journal,* 2012. 12(11): 3163–3173.
29. Weissburg, M. Waterborne chemical communication: Stimulus dispersal dynamics and orientation strategies in crustaceans, in *Chemical Communication in Crustaceans,* T. Breithaupt and Thiel, M. Editors. 2011, New York, NY: Springer. pp. 63–83.
30. Koehl, M.A.R. The fluid mechanics of arthropod sniffing in turbulent odor plumes. *Chemical Senses,* 2006. 31(2): 93–105.

31. Gardiner, J.M. and Atema, J. The function of bilateral odor arrival time differences in olfactory orientation of sharks. *Current Biology*, 2010. 20(13): 1187–1191.
32. Weissburg, M.J. and Zimmer-Faust, R.K. Life and death in moving fluids: Hydrodynamic effects on chemosensory-mediated predation. *Ecology*, 1993. 74(5): 1428–1443.
33. Dittman, A. and Quinn, T. Homing in Pacific salmon: Mechanisms and ecological basis. *Journal of Experimental Biology*, 1996. 199(1): 83–91.
34. Stowell, W.R. Method of Creating an Electric Field for Shark Repellent. U.S. Patent Office. 1980. U.S. Patent #4211980A.
35. Huveneers, C.R., Rogers, P.J., Semmens, J., Beckmann, C., Kock, A.A., Page, B., and Goldsworthy, S.D. Effects of the shark shield electric deterrent on the behaviour of white sharks (*Carcharodon carcharias*), in *SARDI Publication No. F2012/000123-1 SARDI Research Report Series No. 632*. 2012.
36. Meyer, C.G., Holland, K.N., and Papastamatiou, Y.P. Sharks can detect changes in the geomagnetic field. *Journal of the Royal Society Interface*, 2005. 2(2): 129–130.
37. Colman, J.G. A review of the biology and ecology of the whale shark. *Journal of Fish Biology*, 1997. 51(6): 1219–1234.
38. Eckert, S.A. and Stewart, B.S. Telemetry and satellite tracking of whale sharks, *Rhincodon typus*, in the Sea of Cortez, Mexico, and the North Pacific Ocean. *Environmental Biology of Fishes*, 2001. 60(1): 299–308.
39. Bonfil, R., Meyer, M., Scholl, M.C., Johnson, R., O'Brien, S., Oosthuizen, H., Swanson, S., Kotze, D., and Paterson, M. Transoceanic migration, spatial dynamics, and population linkages of white sharks. *Science*, 2005. 310(5745): 100–103.
40. Papi, F., Liew, H.C., Luschi, P., and Chan, E.H., Long-range migratory travel of a green turtle tracked by satellite: Evidence for navigational ability in the open sea. *Marine Biology*, 1995. 122(2): 171–175.
41. Lohmann, K.J. and Lohmann, C.M.F. Detection of magnetic field intensity by sea turtles. *Nature*, 1996. 380(6569): 59–61.
42. Cain, S.D., Boles, L.C., Wang, J.H., and Lohmann, K.J. Magnetic orientation and navigation in marine turtles, lobsters, and molluscs: Concepts and conundrums. *Integrative and Comparative Biology*, 2005. 45(3): 539–546.
43. Boles, L.C. and Lohmann, K.J. True navigation and magnetic maps in spiny lobsters. *Nature*, 2003. 421(6918): 60–63.
44. Johnsen, S. and Lohmann, K.J. Magnetoreception in animals. *Physics Today*, 2008. 61(3): 29–35.
45. Walker, M.M., Dennis, T.E., and Kirschvink, J.L. The magnetic sense and its use in long-distance navigation by animals. *Current Opinion in Neurobiology*, 2002. 12(6): 735–744.
46. Walker, M.M. A model for encoding of magnetic field intensity by magnetite-based magnetoreceptor cells. *Journal of Theoretical Biology*, 2008. 250(1): 85–91.

Chapter 10 Stealth and show
A mind game

For those of us who go diving, surfing, or swimming, having a close encounter with a man-eating great white shark seems pretty remote. Although for many in the diving and surfing fraternity of South Africa, California, Southern Australia, and New Zealand, where they regularly visit to dine on the local seal population, the likelihood of an encounter is never far from one's mind. The rare attack on a human has prompted the search for a deterrent. Previously, we described the Shark Shield in Chapter 9; a device that gives off a pulsed electrical field that can be detected by the shark and that is purported to be repulsive to it. Is there another strategy? Can we move about unnoticed? What can we do to promote stealth? The opportunity to go unnoticed by marine life, besides avoiding shark attack, would have other advantages, particularly for the underwater photographer or spearfisher who likes to get close to their subjects or prey.

Although we see with our eyes, it is our brain that interprets the photonic data from our retinas. Thus, the key to "stealth" is to deceive your enemy, prey, or photographic subject into thinking that you are something different from your reality or to exploit a weakness in their sensory devices. Either they do not notice you or make wrong predictions about your behavior and strength, and act inappropriately. This allows you to escape, take aim (with camera), or defend yourself in an unexpected manner. All senses can be deceived, so there are many ways of camouflaging, or of spreading alarm and confusion among your foes or targets: it is a mind game.

Camouflage is a stealth technique that can involve mimicry of other organisms or things. One common concept of camouflage is imitation of the surroundings, otherwise known as *protective resemblance* or hiding while in plain sight. A number of slow-moving soft-bodied animals are wonderfully hidden by adopting the shapes and colors of their surroundings [1]. Animals living on a muddy or sandy bottom can partially bury themselves, thus obliterating one of the most obvious cues to their existence—their shape or outline (Figure 10.1). Animals may also taper at their edges so that they can form a smooth surface blending with the substrate when they press themselves into it, leaving no shadow line (Figure 10.2). They can also have elements of their coloration extending across the body in such a way that they break up their outline [2] (Figure 10.3).

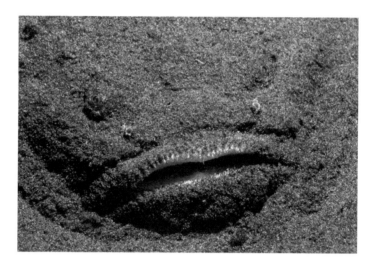

Figure 10.1 The head of a New Zealand stargazer or monkfish lying in ambush in the sand in a bay north of Auckland. Not sure which of the two New Zealand species this one is for obvious reasons. (Photo by Iain A. Anderson.)

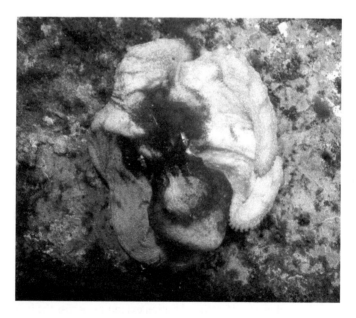

Figure 10.2 An octopus maintaining a flat profile on a rock face in Leigh, New Zealand. The red blotches on the octopus body match the algae growing on the rock face. (Photo by Iain A. Anderson.)

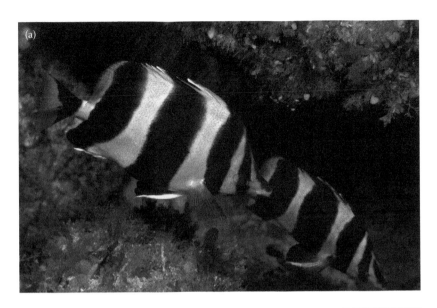

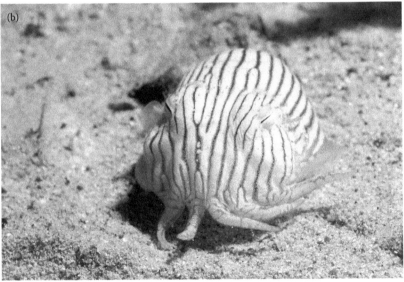

Figure 10.3 (a) The vertical bands on two Lord Howe coral fish (*Amphichaetodon howensis*), photographed at the Poor Knights Islands and (b) the longitudinal bands on a South Australian striped pyjama squid (bottom) (*Sepioloidea lineolata*, actually a cuttlefish and suspected to be poisonous) break up body outline. (Photos by Iain A. Anderson.)

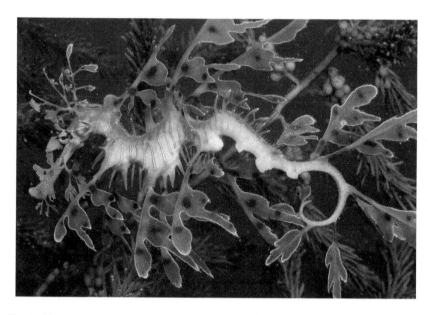

Figure 10.4 A South Australian leafy seadragon (*Phycodurus eques*) photographed in and among weeds in Edithburgh, South Australia. (Photo by Iain A. Anderson.)

Some of the most impressive examples of passive camouflage live among seaweed. An example is the South Australian leafy seadragon (*Phycodurus eques*), a relative of the sea horse or pipefish (Figure 10.4). The seadragon is decorated with luxuriant outgrowths that closely resemble seaweed fronds in color and texture. Away from the weed these fish are instantly visible, but their resemblance to plant structures makes them pretty much invisible when they swim in their natural surroundings.

Another basic component of camouflage is countershading (Figure 10.5). This destroys the perception of solidity of an object by neutralizing light and shade. Those parts of the object normally well-lit (dorsal) are darkened, and the unlit parts (ventral) made lighter. The object then looks flat when observed from the side, and it is difficult to tell how big it is or how far away. It is a very common form of camouflage for fish that live in the open ocean, such as sharks, mackerel, and tuna. Countershading was recognized by Thayer, an American artist, who discoursed upon his findings in *Concealing Coloration in the Animal Kingdom: An Exposition of the Laws of Disguise Through Color and Pattern; Being a Summary of Abbott H. Thayer's Disclosures* in the early part of the last century. He was the first person to publish the idea (in 1896), though an English zoologist, E.B. Poulton, had the same idea some years earlier but never announced it formally [3].

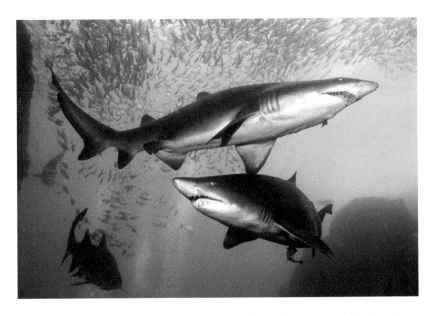

Figure 10.5 Two Australian gray nurse sharks (*Carcharias taurus*) at the South West Rocks, New South Wales, displaying their countershaded bodies that are dark on the top and white underneath. This makes photography difficult: producing a correct exposure for the top surface and water background without overexposing the white belly. (Photo by Iain A. Anderson.)

Countershading is also used as a camouflage technique by the military, making objects such as guns and fighter aircraft more difficult to see, although the effect is nowhere near as subtle as in nature.

In addition to countershading, some fish (Figure 10.6) that swim in the upper part of the ocean, where the sunlight penetrates significantly, have mirror-like skin [4]. Mirrors would not work as a camouflage mechanism on land where the light field is complex. However in water, if a fish can reconstruct the color and pattern of its background it will effectively disappear. A flat mirror in the horizontal plane does not work: when looked at from above it will reflect the sky; when looked at from below it will reflect darkness. Either way it stands out against its background. But a mirror suspended vertically will look dark when viewed from above and silvery when viewed from below and so seems transparent or nonexistent. The fish achieves the same sleight of sight with reflecting platelets of guanine in the scales that are arranged vertically. They generate the plane of a vertical mirror independently of the shape of the section of the body.

The best way to avoid being noticed is to be undetectable not only visually but also acoustically. The importance of keeping quiet is illustrated by the killer whale,

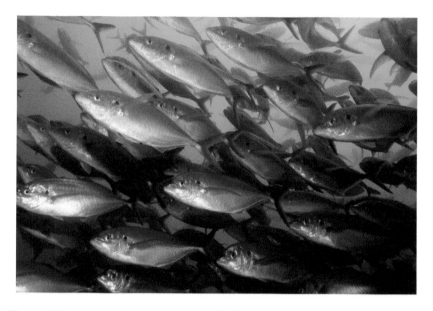

Figure 10.6 A school of mirror body trevally (*Caranx georgianus*) photographed about 2 meters from the surface in the Poor Knights Islands. (Photo by Iain A. Anderson.)

Orcinus orca, a pack-hunting cetacean. The orca of the northwestern Pacific can be divided into two groups: those that are resident to a region and visiting transients. Residents that feed on fish communicate with each other during hunting. Their fish prey are not able to hear the high-frequency calls of the orca. The transients that feed on marine mammals such as seals keep quiet prior to a kill only to celebrate noisily afterwards [5]. For divers, acoustic stealth has been realized with the use of rebreathers that dramatically reduce the sounds emitted by normal SCUBA. For other creatures acoustic invisibility has more to do with not being seen on the sonar of marine mammal predators such as dolphin or orca. In tuna, the loss of the swim bladder, not only allows them to change depth without having to worry about the effects of pressure, but also makes them far less "visible" to dolphin sonar.

Some planktonic creatures (e.g., pelagic marine organisms such as jellyfish), ctenophores (comb jellies), and many larval forms or parts of animals (e.g., the cornea of the eye) are translucent and therefore almost invisible. Near translucent plankton can be easily seen if viewed at an angle where refracted sunlight causes the animal to glow; a method that can be used by the underwater photographer to highlight the animal in open water (Figure 10.7). A translucent object does not reflect, scatter, or absorb light. But the variations in animal tissue with all its cells, fibers, nuclei, nerves, and membranes might be expected to be very visible. What

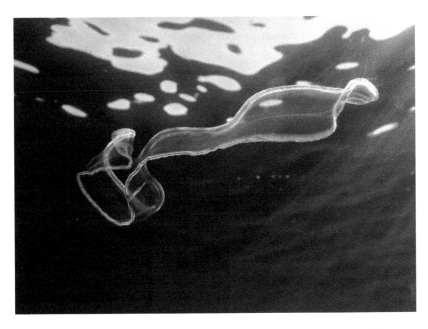

Figure 10.7 This venus girdle (*Cestum veneris*), drifting past the Poor Knights Islands, is a comb jelly or ctenophore. It is almost invisible unless one photographs it at an angle, so that the animal "lights up" from the refracted light of the sun. (Photo by Iain A. Anderson.)

to do about this? The distribution and size of the components are most important; refractive index is less important, and the shape of the components is least important. Thus, if a cell requires a certain volume of fat for its survival but must scatter as little light as possible, it divides the fat into droplets whose size is significantly different from the wavelength of the incident light. Lots of small droplets is good; slightly worse is a few large droplets [6]. Variations in refractive index are not so important. If the refractive indices of the parts of the cell can lead to variations of less than half the wavelength of light the scattered light waves overlap and cancel each other through destructive interference. This happens in the cornea of the vertebrate eye, which is constructed of an orthogonal array of collagen fibers.

This is all rather like the attempts to make a true invisibility cloak that does not require a conventional video camera and projection. Current techniques rely on bending light around an object [7]. These are relatively crude and nothing like the true invisibility of these marine organisms.

But there is more to camouflage than achieving a disappearing act. Probably the most famous of the camoufleurs, Hugh Cott, a biologist who published his classic *Adaptive Coloration in Animals* in 1940 [8], proposed the "principle of maximum disruptive contrast." This refers to patterns that present as much violent contrast as possible. He related animal camouflage to military action, saying "Various recent attempts to camouflage tanks, armored cars, and the roofs of buildings with paint reveal an almost complete failure by those responsible to grasp the essential factor in the disguise of surface continuity and of contour. Such work must be carried out with courage and confidence, for at close range objects properly treated will appear glaringly conspicuous. But they are not painted for deception at close range, but at ranges at which big gun actions and bombing raids are likely to be attempted." This strategy for camouflage is used by octopus (Figure 10.2) and some sleeping fish (Figure 10.8). Recent work with butterflies suggests that too high a contrast runs the risk of drawing too much attention to oneself [9]. Perhaps a better name for this principle would be optimum disruptive contrast, rather than maximum disruptive contrast.

Many reef fish combine bright and contrasting colors and patterns. But be aware that light with a longer wavelength is absorbed first as it penetrates down from the surface. At shallow depths of only a few meters reds are almost gone and a red creature appears dark, unless illuminated by a diver's light (Figure 9.1, Chapter 9). Therefore, if you want to be colorful at the surface and invisible at depth, wear red!

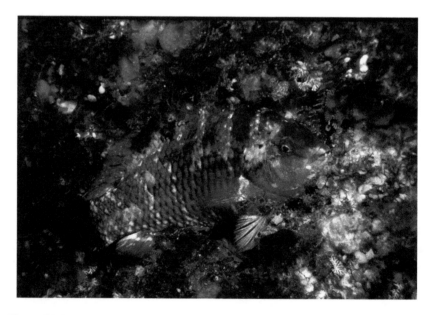

Figure 10.8 A sleeping wrasse photographed at night in the Poor Knights Islands has assumed a disruptive contrast camouflage pattern. (Photo by Iain A. Anderson.)

Some fish can dazzle by reflecting a bright metallic blue or green, which apparently switches off when the fish turns at a different angle to the light, leaving you wondering where it has gone [10]. We see this in our daily lives with dispersive physical colors produced by diffraction of light by close-ruled gratings such as the tracks on a CD, or thin films of dielectric associated with stacks of platelets within fish scales.

A fish's markings can also generate a false perspective that fools the eye rather similar to the "dazzle" patterns used to make it difficult to identify ships at sea during the World War I [11]. Perhaps this is what the Ornate Cowfish of South Australia is doing (Figure 10.9). With the ships, the lines of paint were angled such that they gave a false perspective and thus implied a false shape. It was possible to confuse the captain of an enemy submarine, who had time for only a brief glimpse of the target through his periscope before submerging and aiming his *Torpedo* at the ship. If he identified the bow of his intended target as the stern, he missed!

Rather than copying or adapting to the shapes and shades of where it lives, an animal can assume bright and contrasting colors (aposematic coloration), which announce that it is dangerous and perhaps poisonous. This is useful since an indication of the inedible nature of an animal can deter an enemy from attacking it, and gains its best effect by making the animal more easily seen and thus easier to avoid. Take nudibranchs for instance, a group of mollusks that lack a shell ("nudibranch" translates as "naked gill") and advertise their inedibility with gaudy body patterns or large fingerlike bags (cerata) arrayed along the back. These bags, found on Aeolid nudibranchs are full of stinging capsules (nematocysts) stolen from the anemones that they eat (Figure 10.10). Since the nematocysts release their threads and poison automatically once stimulated, they do not need to be in a particular type of cell, and are in fact still enclosed in branchings of the nudibranch's gut. Thus, they do not enter (topologically speaking) the body of the nudibranch, although they are enclosed by it. Any fish trying to swallow the nudibranch will get a mouthful of stings. The memory will deter any further attempts by the fish.

Poisonous reptiles such as the banded sea krait (Figure 10.11) also make known their presence with bright black and white stripes. If you go for a dive off the central Pacific island of Niue you will encounter many. Looking along the reef in the clear tropical water you can see kraits swimming to or returning from the surface where they go to breathe; perhaps the most dangerous place to visit for the banded kraits.

Producing poison and delivering it is expensive to the animal. How much cheaper if an animal simply looks poisonous but is actually palatable. This form of mimicry was discovered by Henry Bates, who observed butterflies in the forests of Brazil. He found that butterflies from two different families had remarkably similar markings on their wings, but that not all were toxic. The nontoxic mimics

(a)

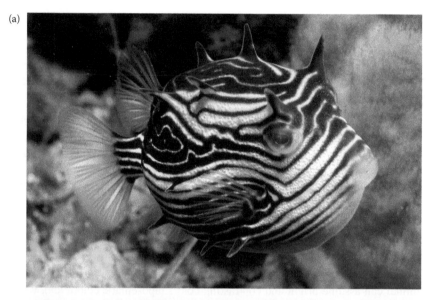

(b)

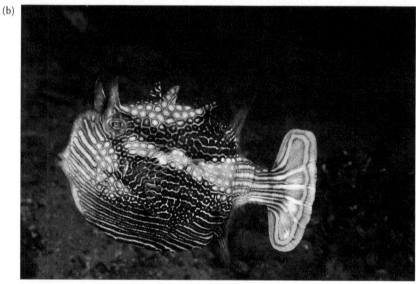

Figure 10.9 *Aracana aurata* (Gray 1838), the Ornate Cowfish. Female (a) and male (b) photographed beneath the wharf at Edithburgh, South Australia. (Photos by Iain A. Anderson.) (Courtesy of the National Library of New Zealand.)   (*Continued*)

(c)

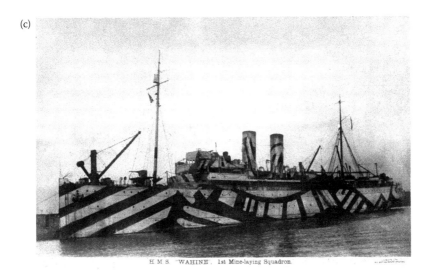

H M S. "WAHINE" 1st Mine-laying Squadron.

Figure 10.9 (Continued) *Aracana aurata* (Gray 1838), the Ornate Cowfish.
(c) *H.M.S. Wahine* a New Zealand World War I mine-laying ship, painted in a
razzle-dazzle pattern. (Courtesy of the National Library of New Zealand.)

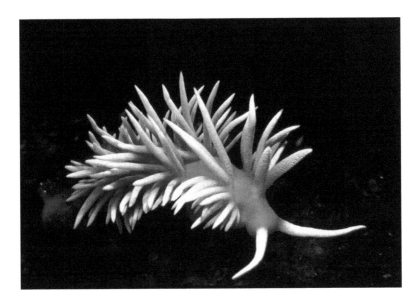

Figure 10.10 The New Zealand aeolid nudibranch *Jason mirabilis*. The bag-like
cerata contain stinging cells, nematocysts that are ingested from hydroid prey and
passed through the extended gut out into the cerata. (Photo by Iain A. Anderson.)

167

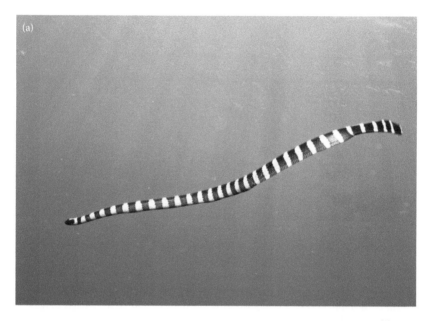

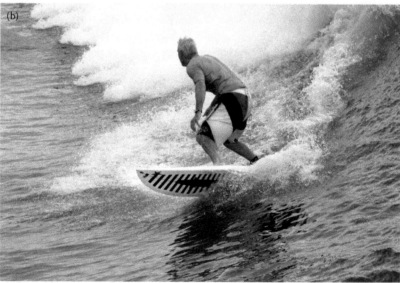

Figure 10.11 (a) Banded sea krait (*Laticauda* sp.) photographed on its return from the surface at Nuie. Its conspicuous stripes might serve as a warning to predators. (Photo by Iain A. Anderson.) (b) It has been suggested that similar patterns drawn on surfboards might deter large sharks from attacking. (Photo by Mark T. Ryan.)

gained protection from predation in proportion to the toxicity of the model species. The more toxic the model is, the greater the number of mimics (often of a number of species) that can gain protection [12]. Thus many species, both toxic and palatable, can benefit from a single warning, which speeds up learning by the predator and gives greater safety. There are other examples of such mimics in the sea. Within this range of mimicries there are many different ways of mixing toxic and palatable species. Although commonest in insects such mimicry is also found in fish; one example is a small flatfish from Papua New Guinea that mimics a poisonous flatworm [13].

We humans are not poisonous, but unfortunately we are palatable to sharks. We could, at least, look poisonous. One strategy would be to use patterns that make one look like a large banded sea krait (*Lauticauda* sp.) or venomous lionfish (*Pterois volitans*). This idea has been adopted for patterning onto surfboards (Figure 10.11).

Some animals can match background colors and light levels dynamically, rendering them virtually invisible to the eye. Pattern control is achieved by fish that can change shading and patterns to suit a variety of backgrounds (Figures 10.8 and 10.12). However, this is relatively slow, since color-change cells (melanophores) (Figure 10.13) are hormonally controlled and most hormones take a significant amount of time to be circulated in the blood stream. They change color by moving pigment around inside the cell going from "concentrated" (the pigment is central making the cell white or translucent) to "dispersed" (the pigment is spread around the cell which now appears dark) [14,15].

Engineers with the Bristol Robotics Laboratory have demonstrated a mechanism for mimicking this using a soft device employing an electroactive polymer (an electronic dielectric elastomer actuator) to pump ink into and out of a very thin display space [16]. One can imagine an array of artificial melanophores in a stealth suit!

But the controlled pigment release of fish is relatively slow; hence, for fast pattern changes we look to the cephalopods (cephalopod—literally "head-footed" molluscs): cuttlefish, octopus, and squid. Pattern change is managed by neural control of colored cells—chromatophores—found in the outer layers of the skin that use radially arranged muscles to control color and pattern (Figure 10.14). Chromatophores reflect red, orange, or yellow. They are arranged precisely relative to each other above a layer of iridophores (which reflect structural greens, cyans, and blues) and leucophores (that reflect incident light over the entire spectrum). Each chromatophore contains an elastic sac of pigment, to which muscles are attached radially. When the muscles are activated the pigment sac is stretched so that the surface it covers increases; when the muscles relax, the elastic sac retracts. The muscles, under control by the nervous system, can act very quickly, enabling a cephalopod to change its appearance almost instantaneously [17],

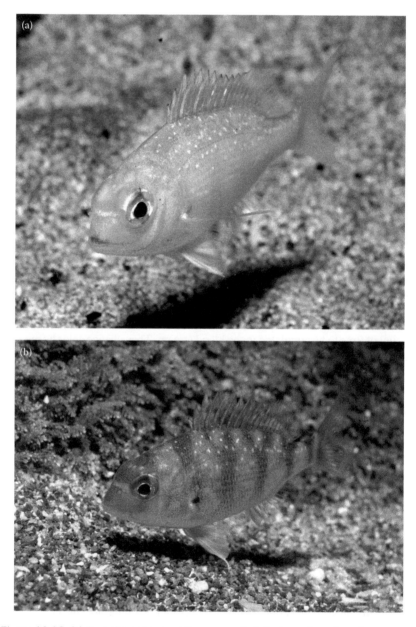

Figure 10.12 (a) Juvenile snappers (*Pagrus auratus*) that are 4 cm long (can grow to 50 cm) were photographed at dusk (a) and 1 hour later after sundown (b) at the Goat Island Marine Reserve in Leigh, Northland, New Zealand. (b) This one displays a banding pattern, instigated by pigmented cells within its skin called melanophores. (Photos by Iain A. Anderson.) *(Continued)*

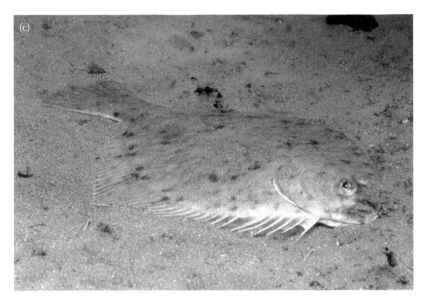

Figure 10.12 (Continued) (c) A flatfish in a bay on the Coromandel Peninsula lying on the sand, matches the colors and general appearance of the sand. (Photos by Iain A. Anderson.)

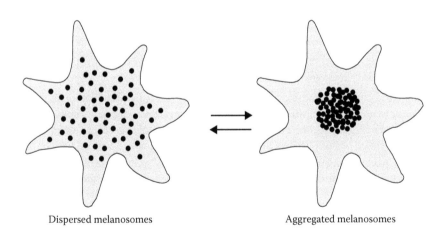

Dispersed melanosomes   Aggregated melanosomes

Figure 10.13 This schematic depicts melanosomes, cell organelles that fabricate and store melanin, within a melanophore. In fish, they can lie homogeneously dispersed through the cell (left) or aggregated together. This process, that is hormonally controlled, will alter the appearance of the fish. Melanosomes are transported along microtubules using molecular motors. (Drawing by Iain A. Anderson.)

171

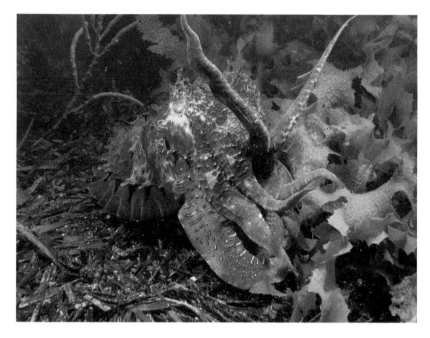

Figure 10.14 This large Australian cuttlefish was caught in a plant-like pose while hiding in the kelp at Edithburgh, South Australia. (Photo by Iain A. Anderson.)

much faster than the flatfish (a cuttlefish can flash colors at a frequency of about 5 cycles a second—not quite fast enough to be able to play a movie on a cuttlefish's skin, even if we could work out the connections between the DVD player and the cuttlefish's nervous system!). This speed is a key feature in some escape behaviors and signaling while fighting [18].

The neural control of muscles in the skin enables the Australian cuttlefish (*Sepia apama*) to assume a kelp-like pose when hiding in kelp and give its skin a plant-like texture (Figure 10.14). Through fast neural control of muscles an octopus can exhibit a range of body shapes and skin patterns in quick succession, which must make it difficult for a predator to decide or recognize what it is looking at. Consider an octopus found in Indo-Malaysian waters that can assume the guise of several species. In a film that was published with a research paper [19] the octopus, new to science at the time of filming, is on the seabed looking like a flatfish. It swims away with characteristic "vertical" (remember the flatfish swims on its side) undu-lations. As it does so it changes to look like a poisonous lionfish. It then dives into a hole and sends out two arms in opposite directions, which mimic the front and back ends of a poisonous banded sea snake. It then sits on the seabed with its arms raised, possibly in imitation of a large poisonous sea anemone. It can also sink slowly through the water column apparently imitating a jellyfish [19]. Each of these

172

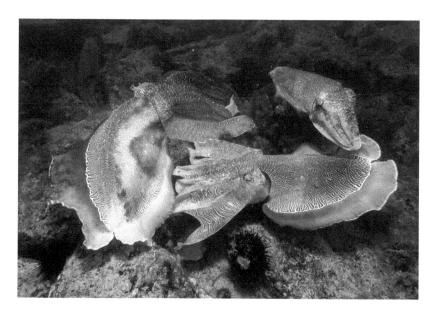

Figure 10.15 An Australian giant red cuttlefish (*S. apama*) in the Spencer Gulf near Whyalla, South Australia. A trio at the top consists of two males having a face-off (the left-hand side one displays a zebra pattern) and a smaller cuttlefish, possibly a female (or male in disguise) on the top right. (Photo by Iain A. Anderson.)

imitated animals requires a different response on the part of the predator, which must be totally confusing. Such dynamic mimicry is seen only in cephalopods and the films of the Marx Brothers (especially the Mirror Scene in *Duck Soup*).

This fast, neurally controlled mechanism enables cephalopods to express emotion and convey information to each other giving them a language in much the same way that we use words strung together in different orders to convey meanings. In *Loligo vulgaris reynaudii*, some 36 separate characteristic patterns have been cata-loged, 29 of which are used to communicate within the species [20]. These patterns can be modulated: there is a pattern known, in a self-explanatory way, as Intense Zebra which is used by some cuttlefish males in antagonistic displays (Figure 10.15). But it can also be used in a toned-down manner to transmit a much more subtle message than "Wanna fight, then?" If one male uses Intense Zebra to another male, but tones down the contrast between some of the black-and-white elements, it is signaling that it is a male but has no intention of fighting [21]. Cuttlefish can polarize the light reflected from their skin, adding a "secret" channel to their com-munications, since fish cannot distinguish the plane of polarization [22,23].

Behavior similar to some of the above has been witnessed by one of the authors (IAA) at the annual gathering of Australian giant cuttlefish in the Spencer Gulf,

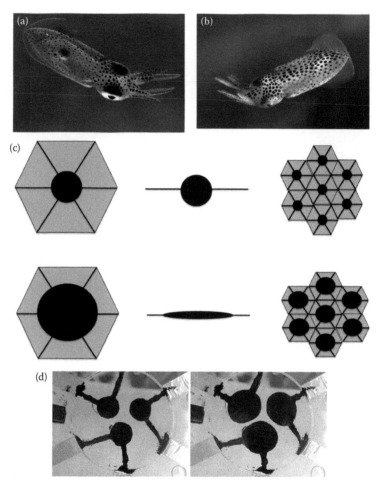

Figure 10.16 (a) and (b) Newly hatched squid, from an egg mass collected in the Hauraki Gulf of Auckland. Individual chromatophores can be seen on these (approximately) 6 mm long creatures in two patterns. (Photos by Iain A. Anderson.) (c) Chromatophore schematics. Here, we imagine a biomimetic structure composed of hexagonal chromatophore units, each consisting of six electroactive polymer muscles surrounding a deformable bag containing pigment. In the top schematic, the muscles allow the bag to contract thus reducing the pigmented area in the plane of view. At the bottom, the bag is stretched, increasing the pigmented area. (Drawing by Iain A. Anderson.) (d) Researchers at the Bristol Robotics Laboratory have demonstrated the feasibility of dielectric elastomer electroactive polymer actuators for use in a biomimetic active skin. In the image, a trio of artificial muscle actuators within the same membrane are actuated separately. When an electric charge is applied they expand in area. (Adapted from Rossiter, J., Yap, B., and Conn, A. *Bioinspiration & Biomimetics*, 2012. 7(3): 036009 [16].)

South Australia, near Whyalla. Each year between May and August thousands of giant red cuttlefish (*S. apama*) migrate to a shallow bay where they mate, fight, and deposit their egg cases (Figure 10.15). Alpha males sit above smaller females and mate with them regularly. Smaller males pull in their tentacles and assume the skin pattern of females to sneak past the alpha males. Some are successful and mate. There are fights between males and this can result in serious biting. The most striking event occurs when two large males confront each other, each trying to look big by flattening their body while displaying a moving zebra pattern on the mantle facing the adversary. The lines of the zebra pattern move laterally across the body; it is very easy to spot one of these giants when they get going.

So, how to mimic this? Again, researchers at the Bristol Robotics Laboratory offer a potential solution: using electronic dielectric elastomer artificial muscles (Figure 10.16) [16]. These devices can be separately actuated one at a time. The actuators are several millimeters in diameter. One can imagine a continuous skin with numerous actuators like the Bristol device. But we are nowhere near developing actuators the size of the sub-millimeter chromatophore.

But at least we have found a way forward and there will be other solutions that will one day enable us to wear body suits that not only provide stealth but also a means of communication from diver to diver. Imagine a suit that will also produce bands like a sea krait when danger lurks! These suits will be under direct neural control by our brain: another step toward the *Homo aquaticus* vision of Cousteau.

References

1. Troscianko, T., Benton, C.P., Lovell, P.G., Tolhurst, D.J., and Pizlo, Z. Camouflage and visual perception. *Philosophical Transactions of the Royal Society of London B: Biological Sciences*, 2009. 364: 449–461.
2. Cuthill, I.C. and Szekely, A. Coincident disruptive coloration. *Philosophical Transactions of the Royal Society B: Biological Sciences*, 2009. 364(1516): 489–496.
3. Rowland, H.M. From Abbott Thayer to the present day: What have we learned about the function of countershading? *Philosophical Transactions of the Royal Society B: Biological Sciences*, 2009. 364(1516): 519–527.
4. Denton, E.J. On the organization of reflecting surfaces in some marine animals. *Philosophical Transactions of the Royal Society of London. Series B, Biological Sciences*, 1970. 258(824): 285–313.
5. Deecke, V.B., Ford, J.K.B., and Slater, P.J.B. The vocal behaviour of mammal-eating killer whales: Communicating with costly calls. *Animal Behaviour*, 2005. 69(2): 395–405.
6. Johnsen, S. Hidden in plain sight: The ecology and physiology of organismal transparency. *Biological Bulletin*, 2001. 201: 301–318.
7. Zhang, B., Luo, Y., Liu, X., and Barbastathis, G. Macroscopic invisibility cloak for visible light. *Physical Review Letters*, 2011. 106(3): 033901.
8. Cott, H. *Adaptive Coloration in Animals*. 1940, Oxford, UK: Oxford University Press. 540pp.

9. Stobbe, N. and Schaefer, H.M. Enhancement of chromatic contrast increases predation risk for striped butterflies. *Proceedings of the Royal Society B: Biological Sciences*, 2008. 275(1642): 1535–1541.

10. Stevens, M., Yule, D.H., and Ruxton, G.D. Dazzle coloration and prey movement. *Proceedings of the Royal Society, Series B*, 2008. 275: 2639–2643.

11. Behrens, R.R. The role of artists in ship camouflage during World War I. *Leonardo*, 1999. 32: 53–59.

12. Lindstrom, L., Alatalo, R.V., and Mappes, J. Imperfect Batesian mimicry—The effects of the frequency and the distastefulness of the model. *Proceedings of the Royal Society, Series B*, 1997. 264: 149–153.

13. Randall, J.E. A review of mimicry in marine fishes. *Zoological Studies*, 2005. 44: 299–328.

14. Fuji, R. The regulation of motile activity in fish chromatophores. *Pigment Cell Research*, 2000. 13: 300–319.

15. Ramachandran, V.S., Tyler, C.W., Gregory, R.L., Rogers-Ramachandran, D., Duensing, S., Pillsbury, C., and Ramachandran, C. Rapid adaptive camouflage in tropical flounders. *Nature*, 1996. 379(6568): 815–818.

16. Rossiter, J., Yap, B., and Conn, A. Biomimetic chromatophores for camouflage and soft active surfaces. *Bioinspiration & Biomimetics*, 2012. 7(3): 036009.

17. Hanlon, R.T., Forsythe, R.T., and Joneschild, D.E. Crypsis, conspicuousness, mimicry and polyphenism as antipredator defences of foraging octopuses on Indo-Pacific coral reefs, with a method of quantifying crypsis from video tapes. *Biological Journal of the Linnean Society*, 1999. 66: 1–22.

18. Messenger, J.B. Cephalopod chromatophores: Neurobiology and natural history. *Biological Reviews*, 2001. 76: 473–528.

19. Norman, M.D., Finn, J., and Tregenza, T. Dynamic mimicry in an Indo-Malayan octopus. *Proceedings of the Royal Society of London Series B*, 2001. 268: 1755–1758.

20. Hanlon, R.T., Smale, M.J., and Sauer, W.H.H. An ethogram of body patterning behavior in the squid *Loligo vulgaris reynaudii* on spawning grounds in South Africa. *Biological Bulletin*, 1994. 187: 363–372.

21. Adamo, S.A. and Hanlon, R.T. Do cuttlefish (Cephalopoda) signal their intentions to conspecifics during agonistic encounters? *Animal Behaviour*, 1996. 52: 73–81.

22. Shashar, N., Rutledge, P.S., and Cronin, T.W. Polarization vision in cuttlefish—A concealed communication channel? *Journal of Experimental Biology*, 1996. 199: 2077–2084.

23. Shashar, N. and Hanlon, R.T. Squids (*Loligo pealeii* and *Euprymna scolopes*) can exhibit polarized light patterns produced by their skin. *Biological Bulletin*, 1997. 193: 207–208.

Index

Note: Page numbers followed by "*fn*" indicate footnotes.

A

Acid secretion, 15
Acoustic impedance, 120, 121, 123, 127
Acoustic stealth, 162
Actinia tenebrosa, see Single jewel
    anemone (*Actinia tenebrosa*)
Active cancelation, 149
Adaptive filter, 110, 112
    algorithm, 111
    error minimizing, 112
Afferent blood vessel, 12
Afferent fiber, 149–150
Allomycterus jaculiferus, see Porcupine
    fish (*Allomycterus jaculiferus*)
Alveoli, 3
Ama pearl divers, 1
American leopard frog
    (*Rana pipiens*), 94
Ammoniacal squid fluid, 74, 79
Ammonium, 73, 74, 80
Amphichaetodon howensis, see
    Lord Howe coral fish
    (*Amphichaetodon howensis*)
Ampulla, 46, 47, 149
Ampullae of Lorenzini, 149, 150, 151
Anemones, 39, 41, 42
Anguilliform, 98, 99, 104
Antennae, 148
Antennule, 34
Aphelocheirus, see Saucer bug
    (*Aphelocheirus*)
Apposition compound eye, 146
AR, *see* Aspect ratio

Aracana aurata, see Ornate Cowfish
    (*Aracana aurata*)
Aragonite, 72
Archimedes' principle, 80
Architeuthis, 73
Architeuthis sp., *see* Giant squid
    (*Architeuthis* sp.)
Array(s)
    of microactuators, 33
    of touch-sensitive actuators, 33
Artificial cilia, 9
Artificial gill, 3–6, 16, 17, 29
Ascidian, 29
Aspect ratio (AR), 78, 100
Atlantic Brief squid (*Lollinguncula
    brevis*), 61
Australian cuttlefish (*Sepia apama*), 172
Australian giant red cuttlefish, 173
Australian grey nurse shark (*Carcharius
    taurus*), 151, 161
Ayre's simple breathing driven diffusion
    tube lung, 13–14
Ayres, Waldemar, 5

B

Bacteria, 20, 25, 28, 148, 152
Bacterial flagellum, 23
Bacterial motor, 24, 27
    control, 25
Baleen whales, 119
Banded sea krait (*Lauticauda* sp.),
    165, 168, 169

Basal body, 23
Basal metabolic rate, 3
Bates, Henry, 165
BCD, *see* Buoyancy compensation
    device
Beaked whale, 3
Bell, 65, 67, 135
    margin, 66, 67
    shape, 63
Bends, 3, 17, 129
Berg, Howard, 21
Bigeye (*Pempheris adspersa*), 119
Blimp, 74
    EMPA fish-like, 107
    floating like, 75
Blind electric ray (*Typhlonarke aysoni*), xi
Blue cod (*Parapercis colias*), 106
Bluefin tuna, 97, 103
Bodner, Alon, 16, 17
Body-bound vortices, 103
Bone conduction, 125
Bony fishes, 14, 106
Bottlenose dolphin, 83, 86, 120, 125, 127
Boundary layer, 9, 34, 83, 86, 90, 105, 112
    separation, 86, 87, 104
    turbulent, 87, 88
Box jellyfish, 136
Boyle's Law, 39
Bragg mirror, 139
Brine shrimp (*Artemia*), 32
Bristle/bristling, 10, 31, 34, 90, 91
Bristles (setae), 34
Bristol Robotics Laboratory, 16, 169,
    174, 175
Bubble-free rebreather technologies, 3
Buckling instability, 26
Buoyancy, 69
    Archimedes' Principle, 80
    BCD, 69
    blimp-like *Trieste* submersible, 74
    diver wearing BCD, 70
    fractional change in volume, 78
    muscle support, 78
    neutral buoyancy, 73–74
    neutral density organisms, 75–76
    ram's horn shell, 71
    S. spirula squid, 73
    storage of buoyant materials, 82
    for submarines, 72

submarine with ellipsoidal hull, 79
sunfish, 77
swimming, 70–71
thin submarine hull, 81
Trieste in Mediterranean, 76
Buoyancy compensation device (BCD), 69
Buoyant material, 78, 80, 82
Burst and coast swimming, 62

C

C-shaped fish turning maneuver, 104
Cameron, James, 73
Camouflage, 157, 160
Candidate algorithm, 110–111
Carangiform, 98, 99
Caranx georgianus, see Trevally (*Caranx georgianus*)
Carbon dioxide (CO_2), 4
Carcharias taurus, see Australian Gray nurse shark (*Carcharias taurus*)
Cargo vessel, 118
Carpet shark (*Cephaloscyllium isabellum*), 87
Cartilaginous skeleton, 77
Cavendish Laboratory, x
Cavendish, Lord, ix, x
Cephalopods, 50, 52, 147, 169, 173
Cephalorhynchus hectori, see Hector's dolphin (*Cephalorhynchus hectori*)
Cephaloscyllium isabellum, see Carpet shark (*Cephaloscyllium isabellum*)
Cerebellum-like structure, 111, 112, 153
Cerebellum, 108, 112, 149
Cestum veneris, see Venus girdle (*Cestum veneris*)
Cetaceans, 138–139
Challenger Deep, 73, 74, 76
Cheilodactylus spectabilis, see Red moki (*Cheilodactylus spectabilis*)
Chemical plume, 148
Chemical sensing, strategy for, 34
Chimaeras, 149
Chirp, 117
Choanocytes, 6, 7, 9, 29
Chordate, 108
Cilia, 29

arrays, 30
bundle, 121, 128, 129
plate paddles, 31
Clawed animalcules behavior, 21
Clupea harengus, see Herring (*Clupea harengus*)
Coastal squid (*Sepioteuthis australis*), 61, 69, 71
Cochlea, 121, 127
Coefficient of drag, 84
Collagen fibers, 40, 42, 44, 46, 163
Comb jellyfish (ctenophore), 32
Common-mode suppression, 149
Compound eye, 140, 142, 144
Concept muscle hydrostat mechanism, 51
Contraction of longitudinal muscles, 50
Control strategy, 32
Copepods, 34, 35
Cornea, 136, 137, 139, 142, 162, 163
Cott, Hugh, 163
Countercurrent exchange
  exchange multiplier, 14, 16
  mechanism, 14
Countercurrent exchanger, 16
Countershading, 160, 161
Cousteau, Jacques, 1
Cranchiidae (*Teuthowenia pellucida*), 75
Cranchiid squid, 73, 74, 80
Crustaceans, 19, 34, 119, 148
Crystalline cone, 144
C shape maneuver, 104
Ctenophore (comb jelly), 30, 32, 162
Cubomedusan, 135
Cubozoan(s), 63
  jellyfish, 135
Cupula, 105
Cussler, E.L., 5
Cuttlefish, 16, 173
Cyanobacteria, 135
Cytoplasm, 50, 139

D

Darwin, Charles, ix
dB, *see* Decibel
Dead reckoning techniques, 133
Decapod crustacean, 140, 142
Decibel (dB), 117

Decompression, 3
Deepsea Challenger, 73
Deep Sound Channel, 117
Deepwater squid-like mollusc (*Spirula spirula*), 70
  model of shell, 74
  squid, 73
Demonstration conveyor devices, 32
Density of air, 3*fn*
Denticle, 87, 88, 90
Deoxygenated hemoglobin, 11
Depolarization, 149
Diatom, 135
Dielectric elastomer artificial muscle, 175
Diffusion, 3, 4, 9, 10, 11, 148
Digital particle image velocimetry (DPIV), 103
Dimensionless Reynolds number, 19
Dinoflagellates, 29, 135
Dispersive, 91, 165
Dogfish (*Mustelus canis*), 104
Dolphin(s), 100, 126
  calves, 94
  clicking, 126
DPIV, *see* Digital particle image velocimetry
Drag, 83
  force, 19*fn*, 83–84
  friction and form, 83–91
  wave drag, 91–95
Duck Soup, 173

E

Ear canal, 120, 121, 123
Eardrum, 120, 121
Earth's magnetic field, 151, 152
Echolocation, 126, 127
Efferent blood vessel, 12
Efficiency of propulsion by rotating flagellum, 27
Elasmobranch, 108
Electrical and magnetic fields, 149
  ampulla, 149–150
  electrosensory, 152
  sensory data, 153
  shark electrosense, 150–151
Electrical shark repellent, 150

Electromagnetic actuator, 62
Electrosense, 150
Electrosensory system, 112, 149, 151
Electrostatically actuated curled
    microbeams, 33
Elephant seal, 1
Embryonic rat heart cells, 62
Eptatretus cirrhatus, see New Zealand
    hagfish (*Eptatretus cirrhatus*)
Escherichia coli (E. coli), 21, 25
Evechinus chloroticus, see Kina
    (*Evechinus chloroticus*)
External buoyancy compartment, 79

F

Festo fluidic artificial muscle, 43
Fick's First Law, 4
Filament, 21, 23
Fineness ratio, 63, 85, 86
Finned propulsion, 97
Fin ray, 106, 107, 119
Fins and brains, 97
    C-shaped fish turning
      maneuver, 104
    Carangiform swimmers, 99
    cerebellum, 112
    dolphins, 100
    electrosensory system of shark, 112
    EMPA fish-like blimp, 107
    fin-propelled human powered racing
      submarine, 113
    fish-like swimming, 102–103
    fish swimming modes, 98
    Froude efficiency, 97–98, 99
    hydrodynamic imaging, 105
    multiple fin ray operation, 107
    NACA, 101
    olfaction, 108
    propeller operation, 97
    reef fish, 104
    reverse Karman vortex street, 100
    signal, 111
    subsumption architecture, 110
    tubercles, 102
    tuna-like robot, 103
Fish's gill, 12
    works, 10, 11
Fish swim bladder, 15

Flagella, 6, 9, 21, 25, 26, 29
Flagellum, 21, 25, 28, 29
Flatfish, 170–172
Flexibility of bell margin, 67
Flexible water-filled elastomer tube, 45
Flick of tail mechanism, 26, 27
Flow field, 104, 105
Foot–ampulla unit, 46
Form drag, 83; *see also* Wave drag
    drag force, 83–84
    drag reduction, 87
    oceanic shark denticles, 89
    power, 84
    riblets, 88, 90
    shark denticles, 90–91
    for streamlined body, 86
    streamlined body in fluid flow, 85;
      see also Wave drag
    drag force, 83–84
    drag reduction, 87
    oceanic shark denticles, 89
    power, 84
    riblets, 88, 90
    shark denticles, 90–91
    for streamlined body, 86
    streamlined body in fluid flow, 85
Forward/reverse motion anisotropy, 25
Forward/reverse tumbling, 25
Friction drag, 83; *see also* Wave drag
    drag force, 83–84
    drag reduction, 87
    oceanic shark denticles, 89
    power, 84
    riblets, 88, 90
    shark denticles, 90–91
    skin friction, 83
    for streamlined body, 86
    streamlined body in fluid flow, 85;
      see also Wave drag
    drag force, 83–84
    drag reduction, 87
    oceanic shark denticles, 89
    power, 84
    riblets, 88, 90
    shark denticles, 90–91
    skin friction, 83
    for streamlined body, 86
    streamlined body in fluid flow, 85
Froude efficiency, 58, 59, 97–98, 99

Froude model, 66
Froude number (*Fr*), 58, 91
Froude, William, 58

G

Gas-filled float, 82
Gasoline, 75
Gas volume, 39
Giant squid (*Architeuthis* sp.), 57, 62
Global positioning system (GPS), 133
Golf ball sponge (*Tethya fastigata*), 7
GPS, *see* Global positioning
　　system
Gravity wave, 91
Great white shark, 133, 151, 157
Greener pastures bacteria, 25
Green turtle, 152
Guanine, 139, 161

H

Hair cells, 104, 105, 121, 127–129, 149
Haliclona permollis, see Western Atlantic
　　sponge (*Haliclona permollis*)
Hamster-sized modules, 5
Hearing threshold, 123, 125
Hector's dolphin (*Cephalorhynchus
　　hectori*), 93
Helical drive, 25
Helical klinotaxis, 28, 29
Helical mixer, 25
Helical swimming, 28
Helmholtz cavity resonance, 119
Hemitrich, 106
Hemoglobin-like oxygen transporter, 16
Hemoglobin, 11, 12
Herring (*Clupea harengus*), 120
Heterosquilla tricarinata, see Mantis
　　shrimps (*Heterosquilla
　　tricarinata*)
Hexagonal facets, 145, 146
H.M.S. Wahine, 166, 167
Homo aquaticus (*H. aquaticus*), 1
　bends, 3
　bony fishes, 14
　choanocytes, 9
　Cousteau's dream of, 17
　diffusion, 3

diver breathing through demand
　　regulator mouthpiece, 2
fish's gill works, 10, 11, 12
fish swim bladder, 15
gas diffusion in tube gill, 5
gas exchange, 10
golf ball sponge and passages, 7
hemoglobin, 11, 12
living sponges, 6
MFC, 16
oxygen carriers, 12, 13
perfluorocarbons, 13
salp colony drifting and skin of colony, 8
semipermeable wall, 4
sock-like salp, 6
Sperm whales, 1–2
synthetic countercurrent exchange
　　multiplier, 16
Yellow-bellied sea snake, 9
Hook, 21, 23, 24, 26
Hull speed, 91–94
Human-driven submarine, 16
Humans hearing mechanism,
　　120–121
Humpback whale (*Megaptera
　　novaeangliae*), 100, 102
180-degree ambiguity, 129, 130
Hydraulic system, 44
Hydrodynamic imaging, 105
Hydrostat, 39
　concept muscle hydrostat
　　mechanism, 51
　Festo fluidic artificial muscle, 43
　flexible water-filled elastomer tube, 45
　foot–ampulla unit, 46
　hydraulic system, 44
　individual tube feet and water
　　travels, 47
　local hydraulic muscular
　　mechanism, 48
　McKibben actuators, 42
　mesoglea, 40, 42
　MR fluids, 46
　muscle hydrostats, 50
　Nemertean worms, 42
　octopus, 39, 40
　school shark, 44
　segment of hose with external
　　inextensible braid, 43

Hydrostat (*Continued*)
single jewel anemone, 41
skin of sharks, 42
soft polymer sensors, 54
spring rolls, 47, 49
starfish, 44, 45, 46
stereotypical movements, 52
tube foot, 48
water's incompressibility, 39
Hydrozoan jellyfish (*Turritopsis rubra*),
63, 64
Hyper-redundant structure, 52
Hypothetical helical klinotaxis
microrobot, 30

I

Infrasound, 129
Inner ear, 104, 121, 122, 125, 127–129
Interaural intensity difference, 125
Interaural time difference, 122
Inverted surface swimming, 92–93
Ionic artificial muscle, 62
Ionic polymeric artificial muscles, 107
Ionic polymer metal composite, 62
Iridophores, 169

J

Jellyfish bells, 63
Jellyfish jet propulsion, 62; *see also* Squid
jet propulsion
Froude model, 66
hydrozoan jellyfish, 64
jellyfish bells, 63
medusoids, 62
Pacific hydrozoan jellyfish, 65
scyphozoan medusa (*Pelagia
noctiluca*), 66
two jellyfish with oblate bells, 65
Jet, 57, 61
Jet propulsion for soft bodies, 57
jellyfish jet propulsion, 62–67
squid jet propulsion, 57–62
Jet pulse, 61
Jet wake of squids, 62
Juvenile snappers (*Pagrus auratus*),
170, 171

K

Karman gait, 104
Karman Street, 99
Killer whale (*Orcinus orca*), 161–162
Kina (*Evechinus chloroticus*), 119
Kinematic viscosity of water, 19*fn*
Krill, 34, 98

L

Lab-on-a-chip, 33–34
Laminar flow, 5*fn*, 10, 85–87, 148
Lampreys, 108, 111
Lateral line, 104–106, 127, 149–150
Lauticauda sp., *see* Banded sea krait
(*Lauticauda* sp.)
Leafy seadragon (*Phycodurus
eques*), 160
Leeuwenhoek, Antonie van, 21
Lemon shark, 44
Lens, 126, 136–142
Leopard frog (*Rana pipiens*), 94
Lepomis gibbosus, *see* Pumpkinseed
sunfish (*Lepomis gibbosus*)
Leucophores, 169
Levels of competence, 110
Lionfish (*Pterois volitans*), 169, 172
Lion's mane jellyfish (*Cyanea* sp.),
57, 65
Living sponges, 6
Lobster optics, 143, 144
Lobsters, 133, 140, 145, 152, 153
Local hydraulic muscular mechanism, 48
Loggerhead turtle, 152
Loligo vulgaris reynaudii, 173
Lollinguncula brevis, *see* Atlantic Brief
squid (*Lollinguncula brevis*)
Lord Howe coral fish (*Amphichaetodon
howensis*), 159
Lower jawbone, 125
Low Re swimming robot swimmer, 22
Lunate tail, 101

M

Magnetic nanoparticles, 33
Magnetic resonance imaging (MRI), 28
Magnetite, 28, 152

Magnetoreceptive cell, 153
Magnetorheological fluids (MR fluids), 46
Magnetotactic bacteria, 28
Magnus effect, 87
Manta birostris, see Manta ray (*Manta birostris*)
Manta ray (*Manta birostris*), 94
Mantis shrimps (*Heterosquilla tricarinata*), 144, 146
Mantle-opening mechanisms, 57
Mantle, 57
Mariana Trench, 73, 74, 76
Massachusetts Institute of Technology (MIT), 103
Maxwell pressure, 47
McKibben actuators, 42
Medusoids, 62
Megachasma pelagios, see Megamouth (*Megachasma pelagios*)
Megamouth (*Megachasma pelagios*), 135
Megaptera novaeangliae, see Humpback whale (*Megaptera novaeangliae*)
Megill, William, 65
Melanophores, 169–171
Melon, 126
MEMS, *see* Microelectromechanical system
Mesoglea, 40, 42
Metachronal movement, 32
Metachronal wave, 30
MFCs, *see* Microbial fuel cells
Microarrays of artificial cilia, 9
Microbial fuel cells (MFCs), 16
Microelectromechanical system (MEMS), 106
Microfluidics, 9
Microporous polypropylene fibers, 5
Microrobotics, 33
Microtubular molecular motor, 29
Microvilli, 29, 105
Middle ear, 121
Millipedes, 32
Mirounga angustirostris, see Northern elephant bull seals (*Mirounga angustirostris*)
Mirror lensing, 139
MIT, *see* Massachusetts Institute of Technology

Mola mola, see Ocean Sunfish (*Mola mola*)
Mola mola gel, 79
Mollusks, 45, 71, 165
monkfish, *see* New Zealand stargazer (monkfish)
Monterey Bay aquarium, 50
Moray eel, 98, 99
MR fluids, *see* Magnetorheological fluids
MRI, *see* Magnetic resonance imaging
Muscle hydrostats, 50
Mussel, 30
Mustelus canis, see Dogfish (*Mustelus canis*); Smooth dogfish (*Mustelus canis*)

N

NACA, *see* National Advisory Committee for Aeronautics
Nanorobots, 28
National Advisory Committee for Aeronautics (NACA), 101
  airfoil, 101–102
Nautiloid, 50
Nautilus, 16
Navigate, 21, 26, 29, 34, 133, 137, 148, 151, 152, 153
Negative image, 111, 112
Nemertean worms, 42
Neoprene, 9, 69
Nerve fibers, 106, 121
Neuromasts, 105
Neuronal delay-line comparator, 123
Neurotransmitter, 149
Neutral buoyancy, 73–74
Neutral density organisms, 75–76
New Zealand aeolid nudibranch (*Jason mirabilis*), 167
New Zealand blue cod (*Parapercis colias*), 106
New Zealand hagfish (*Eptatretus cirrhatus*), 108, 109, 111
New Zealand snapper (*Pagrus auratus*), 98, 99
New Zealand stargazer (monkfish), 158
Noise canceling headphones, 112, 149
Nonreciprocal sequence, 21

Nonreciprocating motion, 21
North Atlantic gyre, 152
Northern elephant bull seals (*Mirounga
        angustirostris*), 1
Notochord, 108
Notolabrus celidotus, see Spotty wrasse
        (*Notolabrus celidotus*); Wrasse
        (*Notolabrus celidotus*)
Nudibranch/aeolid nudibranch, 165, 167

O

Oblate jellyfish, 67
Ocean Sunfish (*Mola mola*), 77
Octopus, 39, 40, 50, 158
    arm, 52
    in bay on New Zealand's Coromandel
        Peninsula, 53
Olfaction/olfactory, 108, 147, 152
Ommatidium/ommatidia, 142–146
Open ocean, 57
Orca, 3, 86, 162
Orcinus orca, see Killer whale
        (*Orcinus orca*)
Ornate Cowfish (*Aracana aurata*),
        165–167
Osculum, 6, 7
Osmosis, 71
Ossicle, 45, 46
Ostraciiform swimmer, 98
Otolith organs, 121
Otoliths, 128
Over pressure, 62
Oxygen carriers, 12, 13

P

Pacemaker, 66, 135
Pacific hydrozoan jellyfish, 65
Pagrus auratus, see Juvenile snappers
        (*Pagrus auratus*); New Zealand
        snapper (*Pagrus auratus*);
        Snapper (*Pagrus auratus*)
Palaemon affinis, see Shrimp (*Palaemon
        affinis*)
Parapercis colias, see Blue cod (*Parapercis
        colias*); New Zealand blue cod
        (*Parapercis colias*)
Parasitic drag, 83, 85

Partial pressure, 2, 4, 16
Particle motion, 29
Pelagia noctiluca, see Scyphozoan
        medusa (*Pelagia noctiluca*)
Pelagia noctiluca (P. noctiluca), 67
Pelamis platura, see Yellow-bellied sea
        snake (*Pelamis platura*)
Pempheris adspersa, see Bigeye
        (*Pempheris adspersa*)
Perfluorocarbons, 13
Perimysium, 50
Pharynx, 39, 41
Photic zone, 134–135
Photoreceptor, 139, 146, 147
    cells, 142, 146
Photosynthesis, 135
Phycodurus eques, see Leafy seadragon
        (*Phycodurus eques*); South
        Australian leafy seadragon
        (*Phycodurus eques*)
Physeter macrocephalus, see Sperm whales
        (*Physeter macrocephalus*)
Phytoplankton, 19, 29, 135
Piccard, Auguste, 74
Piccard, Jacques, 74
Pinna/pinnae, 120, 123, 126
Pinnipeds, 138–139
Planform area, 84, 100
Planktonic crustaceans, 34
Poiseuille's equation, 5*fn*
Poisonous reptiles, 165
Porcupine fish (*Allomycterus jaculiferus*),
        72, 99
Power, 84
Prolate bell, 63
Prolate jellyfish, 63
Proof-of-concept studies, 5
Propeller operation, 97
Protective resemblance, 157
Pseudo-Froude efficiency, 66–67
Pterois volitans, see Lionfish (*Pterois
        volitans*)
Pumpkinseed sunfish (*Lepomis
        gibbosus*), 103
Pupil, 136
Purcell, E.M., 21, 22, 27
Pyjama squid (*Sepioloidea lineolata*), 159
Pyrosoma atlanticum, see Salp colony
        (*Pyrosoma atlanticum*)

Q

Quarter wavelength, 139, 142

R

Ram's horn shell, 71
Rana pipiens, see Leopard frog
    (*Rana pipiens*)
Range-finding, 145, 146
Ray(s), 77, 94, 106–108, 137, 142
Rebreather, 3, 10, 16, 17, 130, 162
Reciprocating motion, 21
Red moki (*Cheilodactylus spectabilis*),
    119, 134
Reef fish, 104, 164
Reflective road marker, 139
Refractive index, 137, 139, 163
Reiswig, H. W., 6
Respiration, 3–5, 11
Rete mirable, 14
Retina-like sensor, 140
Retina, 136–142, 147
Reverse Karman street, 100
Reynolds number (Re), 19, 86, 148
Reynolds, Osborne, 19,
Rhabdoms, 142
Rhiniodon typus, see Whale shark
    (*Rhiniodon typus*)
Rhopalia, 66, 135, 136
Rhopalium, 136
Ribbon worms, *see* Nemertean worms
Riblets, 88, 90
Robb, W.L., 4
Robosquid, 61
Robotic systems, 61
Roboticus aquaticus (*R. aquaticus*), 16
Rocket efficiency, 59, 60
Rolling moment, 80
Root effect, 14
    hemoglobins, 16
Rotary motor, 21, 25, 97

S

Salmon, 148–149
Salp, 6
Salp colony (*Pyrosoma atlanticum*), 8
Satellite tag, 151

Saucer bug (*Aphelocheirus*), 10
Scent, 25, 147–149
School shark, 44
Screw-propelled vehicle, 25
Screw propeller, 24
Screw propulsion, 97, 99
SCUBA, *see* Self-Contained Underwater
    Breathing Apparatus
Scup (*Stenotomus chrysops*), 103
Scyphozoan, 65, 66, 135
Scyphozoan jellyfish, 66
Scyphozoan medusa (*Pelagia noctiluca*), 66
Seal(s), 1, 3, 52, 86, 138, 157, 162
Sea lion, 1, 86
Sea squirt, 29
Sea turtle, 133, 152
Sea urchin, 28, 119
    sperm, 28
Self-Contained Underwater Breathing
    Apparatus (SCUBA), 1
    diver, 2
Semipermeable wall, 4
Sensitive algae, 29
Sensory cell, 121, 149
Sepia apama, see Australian cuttlefish
    (*Sepia apama*)
Sepioloidea lineolata, see Pyjama squid
    (*Sepioloidea lineolata*)
Sepioteuthis australis, see Coastal squid
    (*Sepioteuthis australis*)
Setae, 34, 35, 148
Shape memory alloy, 62
Shark electrosense, 150–151
Shark Shield, 150, 157
Shoulder, 51, 85, 86
Shrimp (*Palaemon affinis*), 143
Sieve, 34
Silent world, listening to, 117
    acoustic communication, 117–118
    comparison of threshold hearing levels
        for human, 120
    delay line comparator for sound
        localization, 124
    Dolphin, 126
    frequency ranges for ambient noise
        sources in ocean, 118
    hearing mechanism, 127–128
    Helmholtz cavity resonance, 119
    humans hearing mechanism, 120–121

Silent world, listening to (*Continued*)
   interaural intensity difference, 125
   interaural time difference, 122
   neuronal delay-line comparator, 123
   otolith-like vector sensing, 130
   otoliths, 128
   particle motion, 129
   sound, 117
   sound direction work, 122
   watercraft, 118
Single jewel anemone (*Actinia tenebrosa*), 41
Siphonoglyph, 39, 41
Siphuncle, 71
Skate, 77, 108
Skin friction, 83
Small crustaceans, 34
Smooth dogfish (*Mustelus canis*), 104
Snapper (*Pagrus auratus*), 99
Snapping shrimp, 117–119
Snell's window, 137
Sock-like salp, 6, 7
SOFAR, *see* Sound Fixing and
      Ranging
Soft polymer sensors, 54
SONAR, *see* SOund NAvigation and
      Ranging
Sonar, 3, 94, 127
Sound, 117
Sound direction sensing, 123
Sound Fixing and Ranging (SOFAR),
      117, 118
SOund NAvigation and Ranging
      (SONAR), 127
Soupfin shark (*Galeorhinus galeus*), *see*
      School shark
South Australian leafy seadragon
      (*Phycodurus eques*), 160
Soviet *ZIL-2906*, 25
Spectral shaping, 123
Sperm whales (*Physeter macrocephalus*),
      1–2
Spherical aberration, 137, 140
Spiny dogfish, 88
Spirula, 71
Spirula spirula, *see* Deepwater squid-like
      mollusc (*Spirula spirula*)
Sponge, 6, 7, 9, 29
Spotty wrasse (*Notolabrus celidotus*), 2
Spring rolls, 47, 49

Squid, 52, 57, 59–61, 69, 71, 73, 74, 147
Squid jet propulsion, 57; *see also* Jellyfish
      jet propulsion
   burst and coast swimming, 62
   constant flow, 60
   fins and, 58
   Froude and rocket efficiencies, 59
   mantle-opening mechanisms, 57
   robotic systems, 61
   surrounding water entrained as jet rolls
      into vortex, 61
Standing wave, 91–92
Starfish, 44, 45, 46, 47
Starting vortex, 67
Statocyst, 73, 136
Statolith, 73, 136
Stealth, 157
   acoustic stealth, 162
   Aracana aurata, 166, 167
   Australian cuttlefish, 172
   Australian giant red cuttlefish, 173
   Bristol Robotics Laboratory, 169, 175
   camouflage, 157, 160
   distribution and size of the
      components, 163
   egg mass, 174
   gray nurse sharks, 161
   head of New Zealand stargazer, 158
   Juvenile snappers, 170, 171
   melanosomes, cell organelles, 171
   New Zealand aeolid nudibranch *Jason*
      mirabilis, 167
   octopus, 158
   poisonous reptiles, 165
   reef fish, 164
   South Australian leafy
      seadragon, 160
Stenotomus chrysops, *see* Scup
      (*Stenotomus chrysops*)
Stereotypical movements, 52
Stopping vortex, 67
Streamlined body, 78, 85, 86, 102
Stridulation, 119
Strouhal number (*St*), 103
Submarine, 71–72, 78–79, 81, 86, 97, 113,
      118, 165
Submersible, 59, 60, 73, 74, 78, 80, 104, 107
Subsumption architecture, 108–110
Sucker, 52–53

Superposition optics, 145
Swim bladder, 14
Swimming appendages, 34
Swimming through syrup, 19
    array of touch-sensitive actuators, 33
    bacteria, 20
    bacterial flagellum, 23
    bacterial motor, 24
    cilium beats, 31
    clawed animalcules behavior, 21
    clockwise rotation of flagella, 26
    comb jellyfish (ctenophore), 32
    control strategy, 32
    dinoflagellates, 29
    forward/reverse anisotropy, 25
    hypothetical helical klinotaxis
        microrobot, 30
    low Re swimming robot swimmer, 22
    nanorobots, 28
    ocean organisms spanning 7 orders of
        magnitude in size, 20
    planktonic crustaceans, 34
    relative influence of inertial forces to
        viscous forces, 19
    robot moves its fins in nonreciprocal
        pattern, 22
    screw propeller, 24
    Soviet *ZIL-2906*, 25
    turning by buckling mechanism, 26
    Zombie powder, 21
Synodontis nigriventris, see Upside-down
    catfish (*Synodontis nigriventris*)
Syntactic foam, 73
Synthetic countercurrent exchange
    multiplier, 16

T

Tapetum lucidum, 138–139
Tethya fastigata, see Golf ball sponge
    (*Tethya fastigata*)
Teuthowenia pellucida, see Cranchiidae
    (*Teuthowenia pellucida*)
Thayer, A.H., 160
Threshold hearing level, 120
Thrust-boosting effects, 62
Thunniform, 100, 101
Toothed whales, 125–127
Torpedo ray, x

Transition, 34, 86
Trevally (*Caranx georgianus*), 138
Trieste submersible, 74
Tripedalia, 136–137
Tripedalia cystophora (*T. cystophora*),
    136–137
Tubercles, 100–102
Tumbling, 25–26
Tuna-like robot, 103
Turbulent, 86–88, 105, 112, 148
Turning by buckling mechanism, 26
Turritopsis rubra, see Hydrozoan jellyfish
    (*Turritopsis rubra*)
Two-module system, 11
Tympanic bony plate, 125
Tympanic membrane, 125

U

UCLA, *see* University of California, Los
    Angeles
Underwater sensing, 133
    apposition compound eye, 146
    box jellyfish, 136
    cephalopods, 147
    cetaceans, 138
    dead reckoning techniques, 133
    decapod's eye, 142
    electrical and magnetic fields, 149–153
    fish eye and human eye, 139
    mantis shrimps, 144, 146
    megamouth, 135
    mirror lensing, 139
    multi-mirror wide field of view
        compound lensing system, 145
    navigation, 133–134
    photic zone, 134–135
    scallop showing eyes, 141
    scallop's response, 140
    scent, 147–149
    Snell's window, 137
    spherical aberration, 140
    superposition optics, 145
    x-rays, 143
University of California, Los Angeles
    (UCLA), 47
Upside-down catfish (*Synodontis
    nigriventris*), 92
USS Albacore, 85–86, 97

V

Velarium, 137
Venus girdle (*Cestum veneris*), 163
Vestibular system, 121
Vibrio alginolyticus (*V. alginolyticus*), 20,
    26, 27
Viscoelastic material, 40
Visual spectrum, 133–134
Volta, Alessandro, ix, x
Vortex pattern study, 67

W

Walrus, 1
Walsh, D., 74
Watercraft, 118
Waterline length, 91
Water's incompressibility, 39
Wave-like motion of flagella, 29
Wave drag, 91
    dolphin calves, 94
    hull speed, 93

inverted surface swimming, 92–93
    strategies, 95
Western Atlantic sponge (*Haliclona
    permollis*), 6
Whale beachings, 3
Whales, 3, 117, 125–127, 138
Whale shark (*Rhiniodon typus*), 98
Woods Hole Oceanographic Institute, 103
Wrasse (*Notolabrus celidotus*), 2, 164

X

X-ray, 143, 144

Y

Yellow-bellied sea snake (*Pelamis
    platura*), 9

Z

Zombie powder, 21
Zooid, 6, 8
Zooplankton, 135